The Optimistic Food Addict
Recovering from Binge Eating Disorder

Christina Fisanick Greer

For information, contact
MSI Press
1760-F Airline Highway, #203
Hollister, CA 95023

Cover Art by Christina Fisanick Greer
Typesetting by Carl Leaver
Copyediting: Mary Ann Raemisch

Library of Congress Control Number: 2016935316

ISBN: 978-1-942891-28-4

Dedication

For Daniel—who never stops asking tough questions.

Acknowledgements

To my therapist, Carole Anne Al-Din. I couldn't have gotten this far without you.

To the members of Food Addiction Recovery on Facebook. We are so much stronger when we hold hands. I love you all.

And to my husband Jim and beloved son Tristan, I fight on just to spend another day with you both.

Contents

Preface

I began this book in the heights of early recovery from binge eating disorder. At just over a year since I committed to beating this addiction, I was flying high with optimism. I would be the one—the only one—to kick binge eating disorder, I thought. I would come out the other side, maybe as early as my very next birthday, clean and clear and normal.

And such is the two-fold burden and blessing of optimism.

As I sit here writing on an overcast autumn afternoon, I can say that while my life has improved dramatically in the last 18 months, I remain a food addict. Although I have not binged during the duration of my recovery, I have danced too close to those deadly flames on too many occasions. Far too many, it turns out, to call myself cured.

I am sure that you are wondering, reader, why I would dare have the nerve to write about my recovery if I am not recovered. I am also sure that you came to this book looking for something I cannot give you: the key that will set you free. What I can give you is hope. Hope that even if recovery is long and hard, it is worth it. And I can tell you that what makes this attempt at healing different from all the ones that came before it is that I am still healing. I have not given up. I have not thrown in the towel and eaten the contents of my refrigerator, not even after I realized that I may have to fight hard and harder for my serenity for the rest of my life.

I am remaining optimistic, but unlike the optimism that has guided my life like a rolling ball of sun, burning me if I get too close and bathing my failures and tears in warmth and light, I am now realistically optimistic. I know that being an addict means that some days I will fall. Hell, I might even stay down for a week or a month, but I believe, in a way that I never could before, that I will rise again, because the only thing holding me down is my own hand grasping the food-heavy fork.

What you will read in these pages is my experience and my interpretation of food addiction, which I argue is a subset of binge eating disorder. You will learn about the role that food has played in my life, from birth to the present. You may squirm as you read of my struggles with failed diets and failed relationships, but I hope that some of you will find yourself in these pages, for good and for ill. The hardest part of coping with food addiction, for me, was feeling alone in my plight. That loneliness led to shame about my thoughts and behaviors, and we know where shame leads: to kitchen cabinets.

Maybe you picked up this book to find out more about people you love who are struggling with compulsive overeating. I hope by the end you understand that the best thing you can do to help them is to love them and let them know it. Binge eaters are notorious for hating themselves, so a little love can go a long way.

No matter your reason for reading, I hope you turn the last page knowing a bit more about what it is like to live each day with an illness that, on the outside, seems like chronic laziness and a lack of self-control, but on the inside is nothing but misery. I also anticipate that the end of this book will find you and me healthier than we were when we started. After all, I am the optimistic addict, and I believe that as long as I am trying, I am rejecting slow, sure death from this disease. After all, the difference between success and failure is merely a positive attitude.

A good friend of mine often says that we begin our recovery from addiction the day we are born. It's a concept that is difficult to accept, given how long it takes some of us to progress. I think that new age thinkers like Deepak Chopra would say that we search for communion with Spirit or Source or our Higher Power from the day we are conceived. Whatever the "thing" that we are seeking is, there's no doubt that the quest begins at birth, and most of us spend our lives dumping "things" into our bodies and minds that neither nourish us nor move us closer to that which would truly fill us up.

I wrote this book for myself, for my family, for my friends, and for the members of my food addiction support group on Facebook, but mostly I wrote it for those sick souls still lost in the food. Come along now. Give me your ear, your heart, your hand. Food is not your friend. Don't think about the next bite. Think about your next breath. Healing is possible. Don't go it alone, because you are not alone.

Lip Tied

For my 40th birthday, my husband got me a gift I'd always wanted but could never afford. He paid for me to have the gap in my two front teeth fixed. With the advent of social media and selfies, the gap—about the thickness of a Susan B. Anthony dollar—became like a chasm to me; a dental Grand Canyon of sorts, which seemed to pull camera flashes to it. If I tilted my head a mere inch toward the light, the gap would fill with a shadow that stood in stark relief against my white, never cavitied smile.

I'm sure it seemed extra large to me in part because of its meaning. I associated it with where I came from: a trailer park in West Virginia. The only people I knew with a gap in their teeth (other than the occasional high-profile David Lettermans or Lauren Huttons) were too poor to get their gaps fixed. I hated admitting that I held these beliefs, especially at 40, especially as an academic heavily invested in celebrating Appalachian culture.

Although for years people had attempted to quiet my self-conscious fixation with "it's not even noticeable" and "it gives you character," their words seemed hollow, placating. It was a gap that marked my social standing and made me even uglier. In fact, some might say that the slight fissure in my grin was the least of my physical problems. After all, I had been obese since age 11. But the gap was a far easier fix. In seconds, I was promised, my teeth would be a perfect line of Chiclets.

My dentist said the gap was the result of a lip tie, or a too-long frenulum. Some people, like me, are born with a longer piece of skin tying their upper lip to their gums. If not clipped early on, the lip tie creates a gap between the teeth, along with other problems. It is obvious that I inherited this abnormality by the many cousins whose gap-toothed grins beam from family photos taken long ago.

In addition to a tooth gap, a severe enough lip tie can cause major breastfeeding problems because the lip wants to curl down instead of up, as is necessary for properly latching onto the breast. Had I ever been nursed, then maybe this slight malformation could be blamed as the root of my food dysfunction, but I was a child of the 1970s and bottle-feeding in my rural community was not just encouraged, it was recommended.

No, it wasn't a faulty latch that propelled me toward food addiction. That would be too easy to deduce. Over the years, clues have led me down many paths, and while I found some truths along the way, I still stumble, stopping now and again to overturn suspicious flagstones, and often coming up no more satisfied that I had been before I started.

I supposed I developed this lust for origins somewhere in my fascination with self-help books and talk therapy, as if determining the what, when, where, and how would finally lead to why. But even if I settled on why, I'm pretty sure it wouldn't fix my problems with food. Knowing the root of my eating obsession would not make it magically disappear. Yet, I continue to pursue those origins, hoping somehow that it would.

Many years ago, I explored the causes of my obesity in an essay called, "Loving the Fat Girl." It begins with lines of sheer body hatred:

Sometimes I wonder if I will ever be able to make peace with my body. If I will ever be able to appreciate it for all its bumps and bulges and disproportions. I want to love every inch of it, but I often come away from a full-length mirror with more than hatred for its far-from-the-middle appearance. It is not that I am always disgusted by this mass of flesh that I try to hide beneath layers of clothing and tight-fitting girdles. In fact, I often feel sympathetic for all that it has been through over the years: starvation diets, brief bouts of bulimic-like binging and purging, constant aerobic exercises, cellophane wraps, harsh chemical diet pills, and a number of other caustic methods for getting the pounds off. Yet, even as I write this, I look down at my thigh flesh spread wide across my office chair and wish that the fat could be trimmed off with a carving knife, leaving only muscle and bone to fill the space inside my skin.

None of the reasons I uncovered during that writing—metabolic sensitivity, protection from potential sexual harassment, and so on—seemed right to me. What I didn't realize then—a full decade ago—was that being fat was not the problem. Food was not the problem. Lack of self-love was the problem. Compulsive, addictive behavior was the problem. Food was merely the tool I was misusing to fill the seemingly unquenchable void in my life, but as compulsive eating writer, Geneen Roth, has said, "We don't want to eat hot fudge sundaes as much as we want our lives to be hot fudge sundaes."

~~~~~~

One of the earliest family stories about me was that I learned to walk by striving for a bowl of green Jell-O that my Grandma Jean held out for me. But my problems with food began long before I took those first wobbly steps. A picture of me taken around nine months of age had appeared in the local newspaper to announce my first birthday. Everything on my little body was round: my head, my thighs, and my chest. Clearly, I was well fed, perhaps overfed, which was not at all how my life began.

At the time I was conceived, my mother was unmarried, unemployed, and living in a two-bedroom house with my aunt and her four children next to a municipal dump in a rural town in northern West Virginia. Combined, the sisters had less than nothing and burned tires from the dump in the winter to say warm. The tires would fill the drafty shack with black smoke and enough heat to force them out into the snowy yard in their underwear. But humans are hearty creatures, and I survived, tucked neatly inside my mother's thin frame while she lived on fried potatoes, wild game, and potted meat. From the time I was an embryo, it was feast or famine, but mostly the latter.

And this continued after my mother met the man who would become my step-father. Since my biological father refused to acknowledge his paternity, an intransigence made even more curious given that his brother was married to my mother's sister, my step-father was the only dad I ever knew. Although I believe I was born with a propensity toward addiction, there is no doubt that a great deal of my dysfunctional eating behaviors were learned at the table with this man, who was fighting demons of his own.

Growing up, we celebrated every occasion and grieved every loss with food, which is not so different from many people around the world. But what was different was the frequency and quantity of such family binges. In fact, whenever the money was good, every meal was an opportunity to overeat. I remember weeknight dinners of two homemade hamburgers and a platter of French fries each. Friday nights with pizza—eight slices each. Sundays of BLTs with seemingly endless mayo and bacon piled high on toasted white bread. As poor as we were, an overabundance of rich, fattening food filled our table until the money ran out and the cabinets were empty. I also remember many meals of government cheese and ketchup sandwiches and endless days of Twinkies and cookies that my dad brought home from work when the vending machine in the lunchroom broke. We'd be redeemed, of course, when we had another monetary windfall. Evenings of restaurant steak as thick as two decks of cards after hitting the lottery. All-we-could-eat seafood buffets after winning at poker. Buckets of KFC extra crispy chicken after the income tax refund arrived. Every bounty was a good time for bingeing.

We looked forward to these food orgies and ate like we'd never have food like this again. Unfortunately, I internalized this message, and it became my mantra for most foods: "Eat it all now. It might be all you'll ever get." And, yes, this extended into the rest of my comforts: love, happiness, self-esteem.

I don't blame my dad for passing on this cruel disease. After all, he is as much a victim of it as I am, maybe more. Instead, I have tried to understand and change those early messages and habits by uncovering them one by one and replacing them with new, positive mantras: "There is enough." "YOU are enough."

I was five months into intensive recovery from Binge Eating Disorder (BED) when I sat down in the dentist's chair to have plastic applied to both sides of the gap in between my teeth, and it has become, in a sense, symbolic of my recovery journey. Although the procedure filled the gap on the surface, I still feel it. I feel it every time I use my tongue to work loose an errant piece of food. I feel it every time I attempt to tuck my bottom lip into the gap that used to be there, finding the spot already filled.

Like that dental patch, the gaping hole in my psyche has been covered over. At 75 pounds lost, I look like I have been cured, but I know that the scab is still there, and like the plastic between my teeth, can easily be torn away by a poor decision, like ripping into a piece of hard French bread and failing to be grateful. I have nightmares, sometimes, that the gap is back and bigger than ever, but I realize when I wake up that fearing a day that may never come is a waste of time and energy. Instead, I choose to live my life one day at a time. One bite at a time. For me, there is no other way.

I spent so many days of my pre-recovery life dwelling on the past and attempting to live in the future. For those 28 years, food was my drug. Food saved me from feeling rejected. Food rescued me from heartbreak and neglect. But like all security blankets, its time had come. Once I started the long process of letting go, my world became large and filled with light. I realized that the THING I had been desperately seeking did not exist and never would. I was hiding in the food and running from myself. And it turns out that sitting with my feelings, allowing the sadness and anger to wash over me, did not kill me, but as sure as I am sitting here, I know that the food would have.

As I continue on in my recovery, the scab over that gaping hole grows thinner, allowing me to move further and further away from the fear of failure that I have lived with for so long. I will not fail at this because "one swallow doesn't make a summer," and tomorrow does not exist. Only today. Only this moment. And at this moment, I am not bingeing on food, nor am I compulsively thinking about food. In this moment, right at this moment, I am thinking about my breath flowing gently in and out of my lungs, my chest rising and falling with each inhale and exhale, and knowing that this is all there is and will ever be. For that, I am grateful.

CHRISTINA FISANICK GREER

2

Lovely in My Bones

I remember well wanting to be the woman Theodore Roethke knew. She was "lovely in her bones." I am not sure that I knew what he meant when I first encountered those lines. In fact, I think back then, around fifth grade, I misunderstood entirely. Trained to understand beauty and worth by the media and American culture from the moment my eyes could see, I figured Roethke meant that this woman was physically stunning—slender, sleek, and, well, skeletal. I wanted to be just like her. I wanted to BE her. But even more, I wanted someone to feel that way about me, to wax poetically over my face and form, but I believed that my body—fat, frumpy, and flabby—would never give rise to such melodic praise.

Whether Roethke's focus remained solely on this woman's physical form is debatable, but he never utters her name. We never learn what she does, if she is a mother, a writer, an aviator. We know nothing of her voice, her demeanor. He tells us only of her eternally enchanting loveliness. In a poem so much about the body, the woman about which it is written is disembodied—ethereally corporeal—

"cast[ing] a shadow white as stone." Of course, the sexual suggestions throughout each verse further treat her as an object to be viewed, to be lusted after, and to be laid. And at 11, when my favorite poet's words washed over me like a love letter from an unknown admirer, I thought that was what I should want. I longed for the male gaze. In it, I believed, was my worth as a woman. What other value could I possibly possess?

After more than a decade of feast and famine, puberty prohibited me from losing weight even during the latter part of the cycle. Instead, at age 11, my weight soared as I gained 70 pounds in the nine months following my first period. The difference between my fifth and sixth grade school pictures is a frank tell all of how far my obsession with food had come. My long, chestnut, curls had fallen softly on my orange sweater and framed my still-slender face like feathers in fifth grade. Just a year later, my neck has doubled in size and my breasts had too, bulging obviously from beneath the purple and white cotton of my Pac-Man t-shirt.

It is easy to blame my expanding waistline on puberty. After all, most girls seemed to gain weight during that time, but looking back, I realize that the rounder my shape became, the more I hated myself. The more I hated myself, the more I muted my feelings with my drug of choice—food. I barely coped with the hormonal rush of early adolescence, which was then worsened by the onset of Polycystic Ovarian Syndrome, a metabolic endocrine disorder that causes weight gain, cystic acne, head hair loss, facial hair growth, fatigue, missed periods, infertility, and a host of other 'unfeminine' manifestations.

But it wasn't so much my reflection in the mirror that pushed me into my first forays of "watching what I ate." No, it was the way boys my age looked—or didn't look—

at me. I was unappealing to them. I remember a ginger-haired boy I loved making moo noises behind my back on the way out of school one afternoon. I remember being too embarrassed to put on a swimsuit for our annual class field trip to the local pool. I was 11! Body hatred had already become firmly rooted in my thoughts, but it wasn't until one early summer afternoon that I turned to dieting to solve my unlovable problem. I had just returned from my yearly physical, where I had learned that my weight had climbed to 137.5 pounds. The shame of that number fell heavily on my mind, but I didn't resolve to fix myself until my little brother, who I am certain did not have any idea of the harm he was about to cause, got on his bike and went singing throughout our neighborhood, "My sister weighs 137 and a half pounds!" The next day, I started fasting.

I had watched my mother and her sisters diet for years. With Richard Simmons' Deal-A-Meal, TOPS, Weight Watchers, and a seemingly endless stream of schemes to lose unwanted flesh. Damning words about their bodies rippled through their conversations as often and openly as talk about the weather and good sales on ground beef. Therefore, it was natural for me to turn to deprivation as a source for transforming my body into something more desirable...to men.

And yet, it never worked. Rice cakes, cabbage soup, running from dawn until dusk, Slim Fast, and still, I remained fat and became fatter. The self-coercion would last a few days before, what I thought was my willpower, would crumble, and I would find myself elbow deep in a bag of Herr's barbecued potato chips and gulping down bologna sandwiches with mayo and onion one after another until the pound of meat and the loaf of cheap white bread were gone.

My mother, already an unsuspecting player in the yo-yo diet game, would admonish me for spending days in the summer reading romance novels and eating bowl after bowl of her homemade potato salad with a gallon of sweet tea. Her voice, which would call out from the kitchen sink where she was watching me space out with my drug of choice, was shrill and nearly convincing:

"Why do you need all that food? You just had a bowl of that."

"Can't you save some for later? For after dinner?"

"You are just going to gain more and more weight by the time school starts in the fall."

I could call her criticism cruel, and I did for years, but what I have learned is that my mother was just as caught up in diet culture as most women were during the 1980s, when the aerobicized body was all the rage. Even though she made it clear that her diet tools—weight loss cards and special foods—were for her only, her body contempt reinforced her words: "Don't get fatter. Fat isn't pretty."

As I struggled to resist Little Debbie's and Pepsi that summer, I also struggled with understanding what it meant to now be a "woman." It is not uncommon for eating disorders and other psychological problems to develop at this pivotal time in a girl's life. The hormone upheaval and identity challenges are overwhelming, even for the most grounded of young women. And I found myself, more than ever before, turning to food to ease my pain and confusion, both of which were enhanced by misinformation and the disruption caused when I discovered my story of origin.

Two years before, I had learned that my stepfather wasn't my biological father, a fact everyone but my angry teen cousin Dominick thought was in my best interest, or at least my stepdad's best interest, to keep secret. I could lie and say that on some level I always knew the truth, but in all honesty, I never had reason to wonder. We were both overweight, with brown hair and brown eyes. His paternity seemed legitimate.

Once my mother discovered that Dominick had told me the biggest of all family secrets, she decided to tell me more about it. In an awkward conversation at the kitchen table, with my grandmother and aunt present, she told me, "Your real dad lives somewhere in Ohio."

Two years later, when she learned that my period had started, I was given another cryptic talk. Both messages were delivered by the same person at the same caramel colored, pressed board table, in the same too-hot trailer kitchen with my shorts-clad legs sticking painfully to the vinyl seat of my chair. This time, the message was even more confusing: "Now that you got your period, you have to watch how you act around boys."

I was too overwhelmed and afraid to ask further questions—even the most basic question of all: why? Instead, I went along with it, pretending that I didn't know my brother and I had had different fathers and that I understood why getting my period had somehow changed my relationship to men and boys.

~~~~~~

I had been carrying a slim roll of 110 film around with me since 1985. It had been packed and unpacked as I moved from bedroom to bedroom in my parents' cramped trailer in West Virginia, to my first husband's parents' garage, to Powhatan Point, Ohio, then on to college, undergrad, Master's, then Ph.D. In the remaining months of my doctoral work, I decided to develop it. I had been carrying it around long enough. I guess I was curious to see what I might find. What images of the past would surface just as I was about to close one chapter of my life and open another?

I remembered that there was a picture of me on the roll, age 11, not long after the kitchen-table talk. I was clad in a red sweatshirt and a short jean skirt, and I had bleached orange hair. When I picked up the roll at Wal-Mart's one-hour photo lab, I was shocked to see that I had remembered those details yet had forgotten so many others. I half-listened as the photo clerk explained that the quality of the photos was the best that she could do. They were too grainy, too discolored. I flipped through each picture, laughing at shots of my Mom, close to my age now, drinking a beer and smoking a cigarette with her sister, Brenda, at our kitchen table. A close-up of my Dad, canning tomatoes, angry that I was taking his picture. My friend Karen and I in our pink and aqua dresses, going to perform in our first junior-high choir concert. Then, I stopped, looking over my shoulder for my husband and wondering if he could see what I could see, realizing that he would not know the man in the picture anyway. I paused for a second only, looking at his thick black hair and the strong, muscular arms contained in the one-dimensional 4X6, knowing that I would return to this picture later, in secret. I remembered his eyes, tempting, watching, devouring.

Later that night, I was alone in our bedroom, writing in my journal, and I took out those pictures, flipping through slowly, not too eagerly, past my mom in her pastel shirt, past my Dad's angry shout, and to the picture of me, just as I remembered, except younger and sadder. I lingered, not because I wanted to focus on the photo of myself, but because I was afraid to see the picture of him, knowing that after a few long looks, it would lose its newness, its excitement, its ability to make me vibrate inside. I heard a noise, and I slapped the photo book shut and stuck it in the back of my journal. I went on writing, convinced after a few minutes that it was one of our cats crashing through a cardboard box in my office. It wasn't that I was afraid that my husband would "catch" me staring at this man's picture; I just wanted this moment to be private—mine.

I pulled out the green plastic book again, removed the slight stack of photos and flipped past my past and arrive on Randall's picture. He was posing on the back of a chair, just his head lying on his tan arms. It was a strange picture, one that I don't remember taking. He was handsome, more handsome than I remembered, and I wondered if that was mostly because in the picture he was only two years younger than I am now.

I closed the book and my eyes and tried to recall that day. We were sitting on the couch, the one on which I was posing in an earlier picture, and he was teasing me, again, about having sex with him. I had willingly engaged in sexual banter with him for the past six months, but actually having sex with him had never really entered my mind. Probably, I think now, because I didn't really understand the mechanisms involved in having sex. And, I didn't want to have sex with him—at all. Nonetheless, I found my will crumbling—a little—under the pressure of his desperate pleas, similar to the pleas I would hear from men for most of my life. "You are so beautiful. I just want to have you really close to me. It will be special." Yet, I think, what finally made me follow him to his room was the fact that he called me a dick-tease.[1] I had heard that one before, too, but this time, coming from the man I thought I loved, it was an unbearable insult.

I never had sex with him again, yet I became nearly-obsessed with the idea of him being in love with me. He had to. I had given myself to him. He was the first person to do what he did to me, and he had to love me. We

---

1   A dick-tease or cock-tease is someone who intentionally excites a man sexually but then refuses to "relieve" that tension.

dated, in private, for two years. Many people knew that we were together, but we could not let my parents know. They hated him, and they hated me even talking to him. Yet, we dated, and all the while, he got engaged—twice—to the same woman.

You see, the real problem was that I was 11 and he was 27.

Yes, be alarmed, as I am now.[2] I looked at his picture, a very clear and sharp close-up—the best one on the roll—and then mine, a grainy shot from a distance, revealing my sweatshirt clad breasts and part of my right knee. I shuddered. The sexual tension that I felt has turned into revulsion. I remember. These pictures were taken on that day. Hours later, I returned to talk to him about what we had done, and he refused to talk. My face in the picture reveals the sadness, near anger, at his refusal to even acknowledge that we had made love. That is what I was calling it by that time. I put the pictures away, reminding myself that 18 years had passed since that day—18 years.

The day after I had the film developed, I met a good friend of mine for coffee. She knew all about Randall. We

---

2   "[He] used me for sex, and yet [he] did not rape me in the sense that a person thinks about rape as a violent and tortuous act. I consented. [He] made me feel wanted and beautiful. It took me years to understand that what [he] did to me was wrong. [He] had sex with a [little] girl who thought that she was a woman because her body and her mind seemed so grown up. [He] fucked a young girl who interpreted [his] touches and kisses and thrustings as love and acceptance of the body that others, and even she, hated. [He] fucked me because I was there and willing to fuck." (from Christina Fisanick "Coming Out as a Fat Woman; Or, the Epistemology of My Body." Unpublished essay. April 25, 2000. page 5.)

had talked at length about how many girls we know or have known who had sex for the first time before turning 12. Today, we were talking about the big snowstorm we had just finished digging ourselves out of. I waited, impatiently, for her to finish describing her own battle with the ice and wind, and then, before her last syllable faded into silence, I took out my photos, placing them all out on the dark wooden table top for her see. I was excited to show someone these newly discovered pictures of my youth.

Then, she pointed at the picture of me in the red sweatshirt: "Who's that?"

I was puzzled, "That was me!"

She picked it up for closer inspection, looking deeply into the photo, I think searching for a tell-tale resemblance to the woman who was sitting across from her. Waiting, with the expectation that any moment her face would disclose the "aha," I was surprised to hear her say, "This doesn't even look like you. You look like a woman in her thirties."

"No, that was me!" I said, grabbing the picture back. I look intently at my face, second-guessing my own conclusions for a moment, and then reasserted myself once I saw my knee surgery scar and the writing on the sweatshirt, announcing the play that I was in that year. "It really was me."

She took it back in the assertive manner that I like about her. "It's like you've lived two lives." I fell with a thump against my chair back.

It was me having the "aha" moment. She was right. It's like I had lived two lives.

~~~~~~

Although my issues with food started years before that moment in the tiny back bedroom of a rundown trailer, my relationship with my body was drastically altered when Randall sexually assaulted me. I believe it was during that time, right in the midst of the act, when I disengaged from my body. It was before the beatings at home began and before the pressure of high school body image. At some point, as I lay there, not quite sure what was happening, my mind left my body.

I became a shadow of myself, much like the woman that Roethke knew. No one could get to know me, because I did not know myself. I felt desperate for love and attention. Sadly, I confused both with sex.

Nearly 30 years later, I am finally exploring what it means to be me. I'm learning for the first time what I like and what I don't like. What makes me happy. What makes me sad. I no longer morph my desires into whatever the person I most want to be with, or be liked by, wants. Instead, I'm feeling my way toward my authentic self, buried for years under the weight of self hatred, sexual abuse, and neglect. In fact, sometimes I think that my Self—naked, raw, and unfettered by societal expectations and my own distorted feelings—is just coming into being in my 40s. It was cut down before it ever had time to grow.

Some of the literature on alcoholism and drug addiction describes an addict as an adult perpetually stuck in adolescence; maturity thwarted by booze and drugs. I think much the same happens to food addicts who begin using at an early age. We get stuck there, unable to continue our development, because to do so would require clarity of mind, body and soul, which is not to be had while in the food. All that matters is the next bite. So, we stay there, partially developed, more hole than whole, desperately seeking healing, but only diving deeper and deeper into the wreckage.

~~~~~~

About nine months into recovery, riding in the car, bound for a bike ride on the trail with my son and husband, I caught a glimpse of my hand in the side mirror. I looked again, transfixed, enthralled by its boniness. Thin bones that moved from the wrist to the knuckle, which had once appeared singular, were split in two—there were obvious furrows beneath my skin.

I am not thin. I am not even what some would consider a healthy weight, but as I marveled at my wrist as though I had never seen it before, I realized that I loved my body. I had become, at least for that moment, lovely in my bones.

3

I'd Die[t] for You

For a good half an hour before falling asleep, I would try to force my mind to coerce my body to burn itself alive. I hated my fat so much that I would imagine it sizzling like bacon in a skillet, dripping like hot wax off my bones and into the ether. I was determined to will my fat to melt away.

The next morning I would wake up, disappointed to find my thighs and ass still too big to fit comfortably in my third-hand Jordache jeans. And later that night, I'd lay prone in my bed, visually imagining my flesh liquefying in my skin once again.

This dour wishful thinking would go on night after night from the time I was 11 until well into my 20s. And yet many people asked me, nearly as often as I asked myself, if being fat bothered me so much, why couldn't I diet and exercise it all away? Why become fat at all? Why stay fat?

I was already being bullied in school for being different—a poet, a dreamer, a creative thinker, poor, too talkative, too whatever—but now they had another way to target me: my weight. I was also chided at home by a brother who was underweight, a mother who struggled with her own weight, and a father who had been tortured his whole life for being obese. My body, or rather, my fat, was always up for critique by others, including doctors, counselors, teachers, and anyone who felt like they knew better. They were only, as they often said, "trying to help."

I went on a diet for the first time soon after my sixth grade school pictures came home. They revealed a weight gain of more than 70 pounds since the previous school year; a reality I later realized was caused by the onset of Polycystic Ovarian Syndrome, a metabolic-endocrine disorder characterized in part by weight gain and an inability to lose weight. Since I didn't have money for a diet program, I chose what would now be called intermittent fasting as my weapon against the war on fat. I would eat breakfast, skip lunch, and eat dinner. I gained weight. I gained a lot of weight.

In the years that followed, I committed to one diet or another at a time. My mother tried Richard Simmons' Deal-a-Meal, and I would sneak into her card stash, and make my own daily diet.

My adult neighborhood friend lost a ton of weight taking street amphetamines (speed), and I tried those for a while too. Ironically, they caused me so much anxiety that I ate to calm down and ultimately gained more weight.

My friend's Mom lost weight using a silver exercise suit that she bought off an infomercial. I borrowed that for a week or so, but I found that the only thing it made me was sweaty and claustrophobic.

Throughout my teen years, my friends and I would go on diets together, ranging from cottage cheese, to white rice, to rice cakes. We were fad diet queens. We did low fat diets and low calorie diets. I remember the T-factor diet, and the Weigh to Win, faith-based diet, with charts and numbers and blocks. We would exercise at the gym and then eat at McDonald's. We would cry about our ballooning pants sizes, and then eat at a buffet until bursting.

Throughout those years, I lost 15 pounds here and ten pounds there, but mostly, I gained. I gained, and I gained, and I lost. In order to starve myself, I had to hate my body. In order to look at my body in the mirror at 5'5 and 135 pounds and think I was worthless because I was so fat, I had to hate my body. By the time I was a senior in high school, my mind and body were ruled by two powerful emotions: shame and disgust. While my eating disorder likely formed as a means of feeling control over my life, the twin daggers of shame and disgust took it to the next level, a place that, even now at 42, I find myself slipping into from time to time. They are deeply cut grooves in my brain.

Several recent studies have proven that shaming people for being overweight is not an effective means for helping them lose weight. Those of us who have struggled with our weight know this to be true, but it seems like the rest of the world still has not caught on. In reality, though, I believe that fat hatred and body policing are far more complex than they appear. There is no doubt that some people in my life have encouraged me to lose weight because they thought it was best for my health. After all, 'fat equals death' has been pounded into our heads for decades by doctors, magazines, television shows, movies, and everywhere else we look. But other people have certainly not had my health in mind when they thought they had the right to talk to me about what they believed to be a very serious problem: MY weight.

As those of us forever-fat people will tell you, we are quite aware of our size, and it has occurred to us more than a few times that maybe we should lose weight. Therefore, mooing, puffing chipmunk-cheek faces, making beeping sounds, or otherwise attempting to humiliate us will not make us thinner. What it will do is certainly the point: make us feel further shame and disgust, and sink our self-esteem ever lower than before we walked by.

Meanwhile, food manufacturers and marketers continue to make foods that promote cravings, and they openly admit to it. Books, like Salt Sugar Fat: How the Food Giants Hooked Us, have exposed the intentional ways in which Big Food keeps us in its clutches by lacing their products with chemicals that raise our endorphin levels, which makes us want more and more, no matter how physically full we may be. You see, in America, we are supposed to be good consumers. We are supposed to buy the junk food, but we are not supposed to look like we ate it.

And so for me, it went on. Eventually, I would lose 100 pounds four times. First, in my senior year of college on the Rainbow Weigh to Win Plan, a diet tool that required that I keep track of every bite I put in my mouth by marking it on a chart. It worked for weight loss. I lost 109 pounds in about a year, but I became even more food obsessed. I was so hungry that I was the first one in line for breakfast every morning. My roommate once ate my 100 calorie snack that I had been thinking about all day, and I snapped at her. I was outraged! I used to go out to dinner with friends and eat just a plain baked potato while they enjoyed their roasted chicken, mashed potatoes, and peas. But I stuck with it. People were complimenting my body in a way that no one had before, in a way that I imagined they complimented pretty women. In fact, for the first time ever, I was attractive to men my own age.

I ended up going off the plan two years later while in graduate school. The stress of my studies and teaching college for the first time wore down the walls I had constructed. My boyfriend moved in with me, and he had a love for McDonald's and other fast food. My lifetime of bad habits crept back in. Plus, he had a car, so I stopped walking everywhere. The weight came back to the tune of 137 pounds. I was no longer restricting. I was in full binge mode. I ate and cried and ate and cried. I could no longer stop at one bagel. I had to eat two. I could no longer put my plate in the sink after one slice of lasagna. I had to have three. I kept trying to fill up a bucket, without knowing that it had a big hole in the bottom.

Two years later, after being diagnosed with Polycystic Ovarian Syndrome (PCOS), my doctor urged me to try the Atkins diet, which meant very, very limited carbohydrates and lots of meat and fat. (I have heard that it has since been re-configured.) The weight poured off of me to the tune of ten pounds per month. Chasing the numbers on the scale was exhilarating! I was obsessed with counting carbs and with going into ketosis, a state in which the body burns its own fat for fuel. And I binged. Boy, did I binge. There were no portion recommendations on fat and meat, so I would eat 12-oz. steaks and bags upon bags of pork rinds. I would eat blocks of cheese and gorge on plates of bacon and eggs.

I was also constipated and angry and prone to wild mood swings. I found myself screaming and crying at my boyfriend-now-husband over nothing. As my pant size plummeted, my life had never been more miserable. I felt more out of control than ever, and I finally fell to pieces when a friend came to visit for a few days to celebrate her birthday and my graduation from a Master's program. For the first time in nine months, I ate sugar—birthday cake and ice cream. I couldn't stop. I ate at the party, and then in the dead of night, when everyone was asleep, I went down-stairs and ate again. I got up early and ate again. I couldn't wait for my friend to go home so that I could gorge on the rest of it. In all, I ate three quarters of a sheet cake and an entire half gallon of chocolate ice cream. From there, it was an uphill climb. The nearly 100 pounds I had lost came back, plus 70 more.

This pattern went on and on well into my 30s. I lost 123 pounds on the South Beach Diet. I gained it back. I lost 111 pounds through calorie reduction and counting. I gained it back. I couldn't stick to any eating plan longer than a year. It was as though after a year, I couldn't take the restriction. I couldn't take being told what to do by some unseen force. I had never felt worse about my body or myself, despite being highly successful in my academic career.

4

On Being the Bigger Girl

In the cafeteria one afternoon during my senior year of high school, we were trading name cards for our memory books. Those manila cardstock placards with our names etched in fancy script were like the high school version of baseball cards. For many of my classmates, the more popular kids you collected, the more cool you became. Needless to say, I had more than three quarters of my stack left when I gave one to my brother's friend Roger. He tucked it inside one of the last remaining pre-cut slots in his book and continued eating his lunch. Minutes later, his friend sat down, also a popular football player. After wolfing down his two-day old pizza, he started flipping through Roger's pages of cards, pausing now and again to comment on the names of what I had come to think of as the ruling class: cheerleaders, football players, and rich kids. When he got to my name, though, he asked Roger who in the hell I was. I heard Roger reply, "Richard's sister," and looked up just in time to see his inflated cheeks mimic my fat face.

That this moment sticks with me nearly 25 years later is a testament to its force. I went home that day, replaying his impression of me in my head and wishing that I could stop being the bigger girl, a euphemism for "the fat girl," "the not-normal girl," "the ugly, undesirable, disgusting girl." I wanted to be known for something other than my girth.

By the time I'd become the bigger girl, I was used to living in the shadow of stereotypes of one kind or another. I was trailer park trash. I was a bastard child. I was the school punching bag. And each time I failed to live up to those expectations, I was punished in some way by teachers, other students, and my parents; therefore, when it came to being the bigger girl, I often succeeded shamefully well.

~~~~~~

One afternoon, well into my recovery, my husband and I were in the kitchen cleaning up after dinner and talking about his new driving job. For the first time in his career he was being trained by a woman, and that afternoon she had told him that she had PCOS. Of course, he told her that I did, too. Over the course of their conversation, she asked him, "Is she fat like me?" He said he told her that I'm "a bigger girl, too."

I stopped loading the dishwasher and laughed. He immediately assumed that he had offended me and began apologizing: "Now that I look at you, maybe you are not a bigger girl after all. I mean, you have lost a lot of weight, and you look good. Yeah, I think I am going to have to stop describing you that way."

I laughed harder and explained, "I am not offended by what you said. It just struck me as funny that for the first time since I was 11 years old, I do not feel like the bigger girl. In fact, for just a second, I thought, 'He can't be talking about me.'"

At 5'5" tall and 228 pounds, I was still considered a bigger girl by American social and medical standards, but I had started to love myself so much that I just thought of myself as me. No modifiers. No adjectives. Just me. I was a size 16, and it felt good, really good, to be in my body. My eating was on track, and my mind was finally calm and free from obsessive thoughts about food.

Still worried that I was angry with him, my husband sulked away, abandoning his share of the post-dinner chores, but I didn't mind. I got back to loading cups and plates into the dishwasher, all the while humming and watching the easy, efficient flow of my reflection in the evening-dimmed windowpanes above the kitchen sink.

A few days later, fall semester began. Every day of that first week back, at least a dozen people stopped to tell me how great I looked; students, colleagues, custodians. On one hand, I was mystified by these compliments because I hadn't lost an ounce since March, some six months before. In fact, I had gained about nine pounds in the few months before school started. Somehow, though, I managed to fit, and fit well, into the smallest size I had been in in more than 15 years. I felt good, not just about my weight, but about my recovery. I had just overcome my most recent battle with caffeine, and I was ready to get back into the classroom and regain a regular eating pattern.

Soon, though, the comments began to make me uncomfortable. I felt, somehow, that they were not deserved, but more so, they were disturbing because it meant that people were staring at me, looking at my body. It came to a head on Friday of the first week back. I stopped at the local coffee shop on my way to work to pick up a piece of fruit and a cup of tea. I was dressed in my normal work attire: blouse and dress pants. As soon as I walked in, a table full of men stopped talking and stared at me. I immediately started panicking. I wanted to hide under one of the tables or run into the bathroom and never come out. I was so completely unnerved by their looks that I wanted to disappear that very instant. Instead, I calmly ordered my drink, paid, and walked out, pretending to ignore their leers as I strode fervently to my car. I barely sat my tea in the cup holder before throwing the car into drive and squealing out of my curbside parking spot.

On that long, one-hour drive to work, I listened to the radio to regain my formerly upbeat mood, but my thoughts kept returning to that moment in the coffee shop when the entire room filled with tension. Sexual tension, surely, but anxious tension as well. For the first time in a long while, I had felt threatened. I am nearly 100% certain that I was not in danger, but the cease in conversation, the all-eyes-on-me, revived fears in me both primal and real.

I am vulnerable again. Half-dressed and lying on a bed in the back room of my neighbor's cramped and filthy trailer. He is standing a few feet from my trembling legs, zipping up his pants. Before I can find my jean skirt in the mess on the floor, he is in the bathroom brushing his hair. Before I can slip into my pink sandals, he is out the door. He is 27. I am 11. 11!

I was a girl again. 13—just over the cusp of puberty. I was drying off after a bath when I looked up to see the tips of four of his fingers in the gap between the frame and the top of the bathroom door. It was a sliding door off its hinge in a trailer whose floors were sloping, rotting, and warped. In my mind, I could see him leaning up against the door, peering through the crack, using his right hand to steady his girth.

Most women spend their lives as objects. Objects of attention. Objects of lust. Objects of derision. We lose our humanity in this constant looking. We lose our souls in this constant staring. We learn to see ourselves and each other as objects. Objects can be manipulated. Objects have no soul. Objects cannot feel hurt. Objects have no rights. Objects cannot speak. Objects cannot say "no." I could not say no.

Those few minutes in the coffee shop propelled me down a hole I had thought was closed. I found myself unconsciously seeking ways to hide. By the end of the year, I had started gaining weight again. It came on slowly but surely. I did not binge. I did not start eating sugar and flour again. The weight came from an extra piece of tofu here, two bananas instead of one there, and "just another spoon" of vegetables at lunch.

By the end of that school year, I had regained 40 of the 75 pounds that I had lost. Finally, I believed, no eyes were devouring me. Finally, I thought, I am safe. Finally, I cried, no one wants to hurt me.

All along, I knew what I was doing. I knew that I was responding to decades old fears and pain I knew that I was trying to pad my form to become unattractive to men. But knowing why was not enough to stop my behavior. Although my compulsive eating was surely self-destructive, my mind perceived it to be self-preserving. It was what I believed had saved me for so long.

Getting bigger. Taking up more space. It may seem contradictory to my purpose. Wouldn't I be more visible? However, fat women in our culture are mostly derided or ignored. I mistakenly accepted the widespread belief that they are not cat called. They are not groped on the elevator. Fat women are not free from rape or other violent crimes, but they, we, are certainly not ogled in the produce section. We are not given the up-down when men pass us on the street. We are not stared at by a tableful of men in a coffee shop.

But we are. The fact is that women of all shapes and sizes are rarely free of objectification, of unwanted sexualization.

At some point I realized that rather than protecting myself from the male gaze, I was hurting myself with the additional weight. Each pound I added was pushing me farther and farther away from my true self. Each layer of fat was putting my inner self even farther out of reach. Instead of saving me from some possible future sexual assault, my compulsive eating was preventing me from living now.

Even though my food portions soon returned to a reasonable size, I did not lose the weight I had regained. The results of my attempt at applying an old survival tool to a new way of thinking have remained. At first, I hated this excess weight. I had gone up a full pant size. I cried sometimes when I looked in the mirror, sorry for what I had done to myself. Sorry I had jeopardized my recovery.

But as the days wore on and the weight held on, I began to think of my body differently. I remembered that I did not enter recovery to lose weight but to stop obsessing about food. I had entered recovery to find peace. Most of all, I had entered recovery to get to know me, the real me. I had longed to shed the many personas I had created to cope with daily life. I had done that. I finally felt like I knew who I was. In writing. In recovery. In life. I had come to find the person I had been all along but never taken the chance to know.

Nonetheless, I struggled to convince myself that I did not need excess weight to protect me anymore. Deep down, deeper down than I could touch, I believed that being the bigger girl kept me safe, not because it gave me strength, but because it made me invisible.

Eventually, that's what it came down to: a change in perception. I did not need bulk to rebuff potential attackers. I needed strength and power in body, mind, and spirit, which would require exercise, discipline, and the belief that who I am is worth defending. Who I am, just as I am, is worth loving.

One early summer morning on my way to a meeting, I walked into the same coffee shop. The same table full of men. The same man behind the counter. The same otherwise empty space. I strode in, turned to the table, and smiled. "Isn't it a beautiful morning?" I had light in my heart and strength in my bones. I was facing my fear, and what I found, startled me.

As I looked at each of their faces, clearly dumbstruck by my chipper, straightforward greeting, I was surprised by how weak each of them seemed. Older men in their button up shirts. Older men in their khakis and loafers. Older men in their stinking, cheap cologne. Older men I could snap in two if properly provoked. As quickly as it arose, my rage turned into pity. I realized that not a single one of those men were brave enough to approach a woman. Not one of the five would dare do much, other than say lewd things about me just loud enough that their words might be easily confused.

I ordered my drink, and while I waited, I flipped through the newspaper, quickly forgetting that the men were even there. After I picked up my cup and paid, I walked toward the door, throwing an honest, "Have a nice day!" over my shoulder as I went. I felt self-satisfied. Brave. Strong. Transformed.

As I drove the hour to my meeting, though, ugly thoughts crept in. Did they not bother me because I felt insulated and undesirable, because I had gained some of my weight back along the process of recovery? Did they not pay attention to me because of my weight gain?

I grew angry as the miles between them and I grew longer. I could hear Shylock from The Merchant of Venice resounding in my head, demanding a pound of flesh. How many pounds of flesh must I gain to become invisible to lecherous men? How many pounds of flesh must I gain to become untouchable? Unlayable? Unrapeable?

By the time I got to my meeting, I was so unbelievably outraged that I slammed the car door, ripped open the office building door, and slapped the elevator button. I regained control of my outward self by the time I hit the third floor, but I was still seething with rage inside.

I did not blame those men, or any men, for my food addiction. I did not blame anyone at all, as a matter of fact. But I finally realized, for the very first time in my life, that the value of my body should never be mortgaged for the benefit of others.

5

Hiding in the Food

I struggled my way through adolescence jumping from one fad diet to another, but I always found my way back to bingeing. Bingeing had become my comfort from physical and emotional abuse at home. Bingeing was a succor for rejection from friends and boys and family. In food, I found a way to hide from disappointment, sadness, loneliness, and all of the other hurts that made up my world.

In grade school I walked home for lunch. The school was a short distance from our trailer park, and I looked forward to warm meals with my mom and grandma each day. My favorite lunches were fat and carb-loaded comfort foods: homemade pizza, macaroni and cheese, leftover lasagna. I always had seconds and walked back to school with my belly full, ready to face my tormentors.

I was bullied from the day I entered kindergarten. My peers chided me for my hand-me-down clothes and the wild stories I told—confusing my imagination for lies. As the poorest student in the gifted program, I didn't fit in, and I knew it.

Eating lunch at home also freed me from the embarrassment of eating in front of my peers. At some point, eating around others had become uncomfortable. It was as though the more my weight increased, the less I wanted to be associated with food and the act of eating. In some ways, food had become disgusting to me, and eating was something better done with family or somewhere no one could face me for making myself obese. I remember thinking more than once, "Just let me eat these Fudge Rounds in private."

By junior high, I no longer ate lunch at all. It was too far for me to walk home, so I would sit with one or two friends, or alone, and watch as others ate their packed lunches from home, which my mother thought were too expensive. I didn't dare face the shame of the hot lunch line, even though it was free for me.

This trend continued through high school. I would eat a big breakfast, and then nothing until dinnertime. It's remarkable to think that I once believed that I had no willpower, when clearly I had no trouble fasting for eight hours each school day while my peers enjoyed sandwiches, pizza, cookies, and crackers. It is no wonder that I would binge at dinner, helping myself to heaping plates of mashed potatoes and homemade noodles.

At age 15, I took bingeing to a new level at my first job. I worked at an ice cream shop that was connected to a pizza parlor; a binge eater's dream turned nightmare. I worked there with a high school friend, and together we made our own high calorie concoctions: fried pizza dough dipped in mint chocolate chip ice cream, French fries covered in nacho cheese and chili dog sauce, and my favorite, peanut butter, banana, and hot fudge milkshakes. Our food creations knew no boundaries. Every night that we worked together we created epic culinary masterpieces that defied both good health and good taste.

Meanwhile, my life at home and school had gotten worse. At 13 I ran away from home, which made the beatings stop, but the emotional abuse accelerate. The bullying at school hit its peak around then, too. So, there was some relief when I entered high school and found new friends. Nonetheless, my self-esteem was the lowest it had ever been. I stopped caring about school, even though I had once loved it, and I found myself spending many weekends alone at our kitchen table writing poetry and diving deeper into sadness. Then, I met a guy at my neighbor's house, and for the second time in my life, I had a boyfriend.

I met Leroy one summer night while I was babysitting my neighbor's kids. After she came home, this handsome, muscular blond guy and I sat in her backyard, passing around a bottle of Southern Comfort. I was 16 years old. He was 23. By the end of the night, I felt like I was in love.

Leroy had been married and divorced and had lived in Baltimore, so I considered him a man of the world. I had never been beyond the borders of the tri-state area, so I felt that he was older and wiser. And he liked me. He really liked me.

Before long I was skipping school and walking to the next trailer park over, where he lived with his sister and her husband. He would answer the door in the morning, still warm from sleep, his blue eyes squinting at the sunrise, smiling, and glad to see me. I would follow him back to his room, quickly undress, and then snooze the day away, cozy in his arms. Not surprisingly, I found out I was pregnant the day after my 17th birthday.

CHRISTINA FISANICK GREER

6

The Weight that Mothers Carry

The roads were thick with ice the night I told my parents I was pregnant. My boyfriend and I broke the news to my mother first, as we sat on that old, gold couch in the living room, waiting for my dad to get home from the midnight shift.

My mother, who had been a teen mother herself, was disappointed, probably because she knew the hard road ahead of me. She wanted me out, and she was sure my dad would feel the same.

I had just turned seventeen and was in my senior year of high school. I was an underachieving Honors student. I stopped caring about school the day I met my neighbor's blond haired, blue-eyed best friend. And there I sat next to him, five months pregnant with his child.

The trailer where I grew up was cold that night, like always. The lack of insulation and ancient oil furnace meant frozen pipes and the necessity of covering the windows with plastic and duct tape. Even with the back door nailed shut and a kerosene heater on high, my brother and I shivered in our beds at night. That night—one of the most nerve wracking nights of my life—was no different. I kept my coat on as we waited to hear my Dad's car pull up under the carport out front.

Leroy was clearly sick to his stomach. His plan was to ask my dad for my hand in marriage. Given that my dad was six feet tall and more than 400 pounds, it's safe to say that he was more worried about my dad physically assaulting him than him saying no.

We waited for my dad to shower and eat his late night dinner. I can still see him there, sitting in his spot on the couch, eating a plate heaped high with fried chicken and mashed potatoes. His lips and fingers were shiny with grease. After he handed my mother his plate, littered with bones and breadcrumbs, Leroy cleared his throat, and I felt my stomach drop.

"I want to marry your daughter."

My father's eyes never left the TV, which was blaring a Quincy re-run, and replied, "When she's out of high school."

Leroy said, "Well, by then it will be too late."

My dad's head turned slightly toward my end of the couch, "Too late for what?"

"She's pregnant," Leroy croaked, visibly bracing himself for impact.

"That's fucking nice," my dad said bitterly. Then, rather unexpectedly, he went silent. A few moments later, he kicked me out. "You are not my responsibility anymore."

I packed a small bag of clothes and schoolbooks and walked out the door with Leroy. Although we asked my dad for a ride, given the below zero temperatures, he refused. So, we slipped and slid the two miles from my parents' trailer park to the trailer park where Leroy lived with his sister and brother-in-law. I was scared and excited. Leroy was glum and had little to say in response to my nervous chatter.

We stayed there for a few weeks, then eventually moved in with Leroy's parents—in another trailer—far out in the country, away from anyone I knew. I quit high school after a homeschooling request was denied, and, of course, I turned to my old friend food.

I would sneak out of our room every night and gorge on whatever I thought no one would miss—chips, candy, even raw potatoes. I would be so full and tired when I went back to bed that I'd sleep until nearly noon each day. Between the bingeing and sleeping excessively, which began when I refused to have an abortion, I had grown nearly numb to Leroy's lack of interest in me. I was depressed and tired and always, always hungry.

That spring, we moved to a little town just across the river in Ohio. After Leroy's drunk driving record prevented him from getting a truck driving job, we signed up for welfare and moved into a one-bedroom apartment. We had very little money for groceries, so we bought bags full of cheap food. I binged on frozen pizza and potpies so often that I was rushed to the ER, swollen and bloated, under suspicion of toxemia when I was seven months pregnant.

A month before I was due to give birth, the Department of Welfare told us we had to move to a two bedroom apartment, but my monthly check was not enough to pay for it. That's when we bought Leroy's parents' 1972 Shasta Starflyte camper, an 18 x 12 foot box their family had used for summer vacations. The couch and table folded down to make a bed, and the toilet sat so high off the floor that I had to jump to sit on it, but the stove and furnace worked well enough to get by. We put out the awning and set our old kitchen table out front to have a place to sit when the weather was nice. We even planted a garden that summer, rows of carrots, tomatoes and other vegetables.

The camper looked out on a major highway and was backed by railroad tracks. Four times a day, the train would come through and vibrate the little trailer until the dishes rattled in the cupboard. Sometimes I would sit alone in the cool grass behind the camper and wait for the train to go by on its midnight run. The rush of wind and the howling sound it made as it stormed by was liberating. If only for a moment, nothing else mattered but the train and the damp grass between my puffy toes. I was not a pregnant high school dropout living in a camper trailer in a one-horse town in Ohio. I was just a girl growing a life inside her body, enveloped in the calm eye of a locomotive tornado. After the train passed, I would head back inside to eat whatever I could find and fall into bed next to Leroy, who had often been asleep for hours. I was lonely and hungry for something deeper than what food could satiate.

As it happened, our tiny abode was set up on a lot right next to an ice cream parlor that illegally accepted food stamps. That last month of pregnancy, I binged hard on ice cream cones and fountain Pepsi. By the time I gave birth that August, I was constantly swollen and more than 100 pounds heavier than when I got pregnant.

Although I was desperate to fit back into my pre-pregnancy jeans, the bingeing only worsened after my daughter came along. I ate while I nursed her. I ate while I rocked her on the bed. Meanwhile, Leroy had started drinking more heavily and was spending whatever money we had leftover on booze. Even though he tried to hide it from me, I found his empty cans in the trash out back, usually when I was trying to hide the wrappers from my own deadly habit.

We argued often, and he wanted nothing to do with our daughter, Samantha. He spent as much time as he could digging in the garden or working on his car. Eventually, we realized we had to do something, so I moved in with my parents, and he went to the Carolinas to stay with his family while he looked for work. A month later he returned to the Valley, financially broke and spiritually empty. He took a job at a fast food restaurant, and we rented half a duplex not far from my parents' house.

We relied on a kerosene heater for warmth because we could not afford to turn on the gas. I stayed home with Samantha and tried to stick to my diet, and failed. In fact, I was so obsessed with food that the report I gave to the police the morning after Leroy murdered Samantha included a detailed description of the meal I made for dinner the night before: pork chops, Rice-a-Roni, and corn.

7

Splitting in Two

The night she was murdered, I split in two. My mind shot out of my body, and before I knew it, I was watching myself frantically pacing the ER waiting room. I couldn't hear the screams, but I saw myself screaming. I couldn't feel my fists thrashing my own knees, but I watched as my body jumped up and down in a green, padded chair, my long, uncombed hair swinging in my face.

My daughter was dead.

Psychologists call this out-of-body experience splitting, and it is not uncommon during major trauma. Finding my 3 ½-month old daughter cold and gray in her bassinet was major trauma, and rather than being out of my mind, as lay people call insanity, my mind was clearly out of my body.

We had lived in our new apartment for just 11 days when Samantha's father shook her to death in our living room. A videotaped confession allegedly shows him acting out what he did that night, including throwing her up against the wall and shaking her until she stopped crying. However, given that I had seen how inaccurate the local media was when reporting other known details of her life and death, I am certain that I do not know the real story and never will. I knew then what I know now: my daughter was killed by her father.

I remember running as fast as I could into the street, carrying her limp body as I screamed, "My baby! Somebody save my baby!" I remember giving her mouth-to –mouth resuscitation in the ten-minute drive to the hospital, her father acting like he gave a damn, driving over 100 miles per hour with the cops in hot pursuit. I remember jumping out of the frog- green '78 Cougar, its glass packs still crackling, and stumbling through the emergency room doors. Moments later, my daughter was gone from my arms, and my mind left my body.

It's easy to almost laugh about such experiences. It's too Sylvia Brown or daytime talk show fodder, right? But in reality, my mind knew exactly what it was doing. It was far too painful to stay and feel such incredible anguish. To save itself, to save myself, it left and became a witness to torment.

Later that night, after I had kissed my daughter goodbye for the last time, I stood up on the cement retaining wall outside the emergency room doors. I imagined what it would be like to jump through the yellow streetlights to the parking lot below. How my body would drift through the frigid November air, weightless, timeless. I closed my eyes and breathed in my anticipated nothingness. Then, I came back into my body. For some reason, I didn't jump that night. For some reason, I climbed down from the wall, weaved my way through parked ambulances and faced a completely different world than the one I had woken up to that morning.

In the months following Samantha's murder, I slipped in and out of various psychological states. I blacked out on Christmas Eve and woke up lying in the cold, wet mud that still mounded her grave. I hallucinated my grandfather, dressed in his brown burial suit, bringing Samantha back to life right in the living room. I experienced very little sense of a stable self. I was both anxious and depressed, hysterical and subdued. Somewhere in the midst of my conscious and subconscious mind breaking up and breaking down, a new me emerged.

I found myself nearly crushed with empathy for the world. For the first time in my life, I felt a kinship with others who were struggling. I felt their tears. I felt their pain. I understood what it meant to be judged for grieving in ways others did not expect. I understood what it meant to lose everything in a matter of minutes. Although some people have told me that Samantha's death made me "grow up fast," in reality, the trauma of losing her urged me to develop a grateful heart. I was grateful that my parents let me live with them. I was grateful to have a job. I was grateful to be alive.

That transformation from a forlorn, distraught, traumatized teen into an optimistic, driven woman was completed in the middle of the night in the back of a gas station with my arm stuck deep inside a popcorn machine.

A few months after Samantha died, I started looking for work, which turned out to be more difficult than it had ever been before. Few businesses in my small town wanted the stigma of a murdered baby's mother working at their front desk and my lack of education and transportation kept me bound to minimum wage jobs within walking distance. I finally found a job at an all-night gas station.

Working the midnight shift meant that the doors were locked, and I was alone all night inside. My only interaction with other people was through an intercom near the cash register. Customers would press the button, place their orders, and pay, and I would slide their items through a drawer in the window. It was a lonely job. I was a lonely person. I had few friends, and my husband was in prison. It is no wonder, then, that I binged for nearly all of my 6-hour shift.

The convenience store was stocked with junk food that ranged from Twinkies, to pretzels, to donuts delivered by the local bakery. I easily spent a day's wages each week on food. I stole plenty of food, too. Every time I went into the walk-in cooler, I took a piece of the ham that we sold in our deli, an ice cream sandwich or some other treat. I gorged all night long as I went about my chores and waited on customers. I was in a dead end job, working for dead end wages. Then, one night, my world shifted.

At exactly 1:15 a.m. every single night I worked, Ralph would knock on my window, and I would slide him a case of Busch and two packs of Marlboro Reds. The only words he ever spoke were his order, which he stopped repeating once it was clear that I had memorized it. I only knew his name because it was stitched on his uniform. I guessed that he was a security guard at one of the local closed chemical plants, because he carried a flashlight on his left hip and a fat set of jangling keys on his right. His collar-length brown hair receded a bit from his thin, almost always unshaven face. I studied his hands each time he placed his bills in the drawer and again when he dug out his change. His nails were clean, but his skin was dry and cracked, and sometimes spotted with dots of blood.

After weeks of Ralph's regular purchases, I started to pity him. He seemed lonely, and I wondered what he was working for—beer and cigarettes? Then, one unusually cold night in early May, I heard a knock on the front window. My right arm was deep inside the popcorn machine, carefully scrubbing the stuck-on butter and salt from the tempered glass sides. I looked up and mouthed to the person I knew would be Ralph, "just a minute." I pulled out my arm, took off my latex glove, and walked to the beer case for Ralph's usual. He paid with exact change as usual, and as I slid his beer and cigarettes out to him, he looked up at me and muttered, "I guess we are both in some sort of a rut." I smiled and nodded in agreement, partially shocked to hear his voice, but mostly stunned that he was right. I was in a rut, and I needed to get out right then and there or I never would.

I spent the rest of that night trying to figure out where I was and where I wanted to be. I knew that I did not want to continue selling beer and cigarettes for the rest of my life, but I didn't even have a high school diploma. A month or so went by, and I decided to go back to high school and repeat my senior year. I could have pursued a GED, but something in me refused to settle. For the first time that I could remember, I felt a surge of motivation swell within me. Suddenly, I was on a mission. I was going to finish high school, and so I did.

I spent an entire year breezing through my classes and struggling with bullies. I lived in a small town, so everyone knew me and knew that Samantha had been killed, but I kept on going, fleeing only once when another student asked me if my daughter was walking yet. When I said nothing, she answered for me, "Oh, yeah, that's right. She's dead."

Toward the end of January, my guidance counselor suggested I apply to college. I was shocked. I didn't know anyone who had gone to college, beyond my teachers and doctors. No one in my family had even graduated from high school. How could I—penniless and with very little support—go to college? I applied to just one school, West

Liberty University, and it was one of the best moves of my entire life.

Not only did I make lifelong friends (and even found a husband) there, but for the first time since childhood, I found a place where I belonged. My professors praised me for my intelligence and my writing skills. I was happy because I was finally loved for who I was and not shunned because I wasn't who everyone else expected me to be. My joy was muted only by my unabated desire to be thin. Even with acceptance from friends and faculty, I was unable to shake my need to fit into a small size, so I did. For the first time in my life, I was able to lose a large amount of weight—over 100 pounds—and I headed off to graduate school to become a professor. Yes, I loved college so much that I never wanted to leave.

I was a new person: thinner, more energetic. Some people even called me attractive. My new boyfriend moved into my tiny apartment with me, and I was able to hold on to my dieting ways despite his daily—sometimes twice daily—fast food meals. But by the time I reached the final stretch of my doctorate, my weight had soared once again, and I had become even more obsessed with food, dieting and my appearance than ever. I was in a relationship with a loving man, enrolled in an excellent Ph.D. program, and teaching college classes. Yet, something hurt. Something hurt very deeply, and none of those things could make it stop.

8

Learning to Shut My Mouth

Hindsight is 20/20, as the old axiom goes, and it has never been more true for me than in the case of Binge Eating Disorder. It is no wonder that it took me nearly three decades to understand and accept that I had an eating disorder. Not only are eating disorders misunderstood, but also, with the way our culture looks at food, women's bodies, dieting and eating, it is no wonder that someone could suffer their entire life with no relief. I believe BED is the most misunderstood of all eating disorders because of societal attitudes about obesity. Although not all persons with BED are overweight, the majority of us are. Instead of treating the disorder, doctors and counselors focus on the symptom—excess weight—which, ironically, most often leads to a worsening of the disorder. Meanwhile, the sufferer seeks answers in the wrong places. In my case, my eating disorder was masked by other maladies, including impulse control and Polycystic Ovarian Syndrome (PCOS). Had I looked past the medical community's emphasis on my weight as the problem and searched for the root, I might have found recovery and peace much sooner.

As a teen, my weight was an object of scrutiny from family, friends, teachers, doctors, and society at large. It became painfully obvious early on that my body was under near constant surveillance and judgment. In Western culture the fat woman's body is reviled, as it is a physical representation of perceived gluttony and lack of control. Fat girls and women are subjected to teasing, pressured to lose weight "no matter what," and socially sanctioned. They are told to expect rejection, especially from the opposite sex. Fat bodies can never be seen as normal variations on the human form, but are inherently diseased. They are always viewed as leaches on society's resources and disgusting reminders of excess and greed. Bias against and public hatred toward fat bodies is both accepted and reinforced in all but the few small pockets of women's groups that are trying to send a message that all bodies should be—have the right to be—loved. It is largely due to this fat bias that my eating disorder went unchallenged until I was almost 40 years old.

In addition, I was diagnosed with PCOS (finally!) at the age of 27. No one listened when I said my periods were irregular. No one listened when I said that I had terrible mood swings. No one listened when I complained of fuzzy-headedness. Instead, all doctors had to say was that I needed to lose weight and then I would be better. Of course, not a single one of them ever gave me the tools to undertake weight loss, so I was left feeling like a failure, like I had no willpower. Meanwhile, I was almost finished with my Ph.D. and had achieved many other great milestones in my life.

Left with no answers, I did what I do best: research. The Internet was young then, but I found a doctor in Costa Rica who did diagnoses over email. I sent him a long narrative of my symptoms, and he wrote back just a few hours later with a firm answer: Polycystic Ovarian Syndrome. Two days later, I went to back to my doctor in an attempt to confirm this diagnosis, and he said to me, "Oh yeah, probably, but really, you need to put down the chips and walk on the treadmill."

I fought hard to not cry in front of him because he didn't deserve to see my tears, so I rushed out of his office, sat on the Health Center steps and sobbed for a good 20 minutes. Instead of getting any real help, I was left to feel like my illness was based entirely on my own actions. I was fat and sick because I chose to be fat and sick. Although we know that lifestyle impacts physical and mental well being, there was something going on with my body that I had no control over. And thus began yet another decade of dieting and weight loss obsession, and yet another decade of not getting the help I needed for my eating disorder. I got sicker and sicker with each restrictive eating plan I tried and failed. Nine months of radical weight loss, followed by two years of rapid weight gain. Rinse and repeat.

Along the way, though, I continued to educate myself about PCOS and learned that it was likely inherited and that symptoms of mine that had gone unidentified were directly related to the syndrome: excessive facial hair, head hair thinning, cystic acne, skin tags, brown patches of skin, and other unsightly physical manifestations. It became my life's work to not only educate myself about the disease, but to educate others as well. I joined several online support groups and even held my own in-person meetings.

Over the years, I tried all kinds of treatments for PCOS, including taking Glucophage, an insulin sensitizing drug. None of those treatments worked long-term, and I struggled with infertility and miscarriages. It was during a consultation with a fertility specialist that I first saw the spark of what would later become my self-diagnosis of BED. I was telling her about how PCOS had impacted my life when I said, "I don't think I have an eating disorder. I mean, I engage in disordered eating, but I don't have an eating disorder." She agreed, and we moved on. Later, I would remember this moment as the first time I ever admitted openly that I had a problem with food that was more about an illness than an internal failing.

Meanwhile, the onslaught of my fat body continued. An hour after my conversation with the specialist, I had a transvaginal ultrasound, which involved inserting a long wand into the vagina to get a clear scan of the uterine cavity. The doctor reading the results patted me on my bare leg, still in stirrups, and said, "You need to lose weight, honey, and the best way to do that is to just shut your mouth, like this." He then demonstrated, very theatrically, the closing of his mouth.

Not only did I find myself unable to bear a child, but I was fat, too, and all of this because I simply would not close my mouth. I did not ask for his advice. I did not want his commentary, but it was pushed on me when I couldn't get up to defend myself. I was furious, and for the first time in my life, I expressed that anger. Since the doctor doing the exam left before I could speak my mind, I went right back up to my specialist's office, waiting two hours until she was free again, and told her what he said. She was very sympathetic and warm in her response, but once again, I left empty handed. Instead of finding treatment for what I had finally come to see as "disordered eating," I left the clinic and went right into the bookstore to look for the latest diet book. After all, I needed to learn how to shut my mouth.

9

My Body, My Fat, My Self

Head down, I round the corner onto Court Street and shuffle slowly to the car, barely aware of the throng of students and professors making their way uptown for lunch or coffee or noon-time drinks at the Union bar. I'm in my second year of study in a selective doctoral program. I should have been in with the crowd, but I am not. I am miserable. I am tired. I am disgusted. I am fat.

The power of body shaming overwhelmed me nearly all of my life, but it reached a mighty crescendo in graduate school when my health deteriorated. By the end of my doctoral program not only was I sick and tired, I hated myself so deeply that I didn't want to get out of bed in the morning. The self-abuse had become so ingrained that it had become truth.

Does my ass jiggle when I walk?

Why can't I buy normal clothes?

I bet everyone thinks I stink.

It's no wonder I couldn't find a date in high school.

I hope no one looks at me now that I am fatter.

Was that guy mooing at me?

I had gained 80 pounds since my boyfriend, Nick, moved in a couple of years prior. None of my clothes fit, and I felt like a great waddling beast pounding the brick-lined streets of the college town where I studied and taught. Despite his loving comments and attention, I was so obsessed with how other people must see me that I was miserable. Once outgoing in my department, I now found myself making excuses for not attending parties and literary events. I stayed home. I stayed home and I ate.

In a sense, my thoughts and actions were narcissistic. To think that other people thought about my body that much really reflected my state of mind and maturity. Even if people noticed my weight gain or thought I was grossly fat, how long did they think it? To presume that anyone cared about how I looked beyond a second was self-centered and exemplified how diseased my thinking had become.

Of course, we are taught from birth that female bodies are constantly under surveillance, so it is no wonder that I believed that I was always on display.

I found momentary comfort in food. Being a food addict means sacrificing the future for the now. Paradoxically, bingeing takes us farther away from the present moment than daydreaming. The chemical high alone takes the binger to another place. It cleaves the mind from the body and disrupts reality. But it only lasts for a short while, sometimes even ending before the food runs out. By the time the wrappers are in the trash and the bowls are in the sink, the high is gone. In its place are feelings of sadness and guilt and shame. The inner monologue that had been silenced with food starts up again, louder than before.

I am just going to be fat my whole life.

Why am I unable to control my eating?

Dad was right. I'm just a lazy pig.

Why did I eat all that?

I need to work out NOW.

Fine, I won't eat anything else for the rest of the day.

Combined with physical sensations of bloating, painful stomach stretching, a rapid heartbeat, and dizziness, I paid dearly for each momentary escape from reality.

The biggest binge behavior I've battled, and still struggle with from time to time, is overcoming the use of compulsive eating as a means of procrastination. If the house needed to be cleaned, I'd binge. If I had papers to grade, I'd binge. If I had cat litter to scoop, I'd binge. After all, I couldn't do anything else if I was eating, including thinking. If I didn't want to admit to lying to my friend, I'd binge. If I didn't want to remember my daughter's grey face the night she died, I'd binge. If I didn't want to think about how much debt I'd amassed, I'd binge.

Compulsive eating required all of my energy and focus. It was the ultimate escape. It was my form of levitating. If I didn't like what the real world had to offer, I would transport to a place fueled by sugar and starch, fat and salt, where no one could hurt me. What I didn't realize was that each bite that took me to places unknown was also hurting me. I wasn't just leaving behind heartbreak and pain, but I was abandoning myself as well. I am sure that is why I kept going back and drugging up. I had to keep searching for that place where nothing mattered but the movement of my mouth, the chemicals lighting up my brain, and the chance to forget. The psychological outcome was depression and anxiety. The physical outcome was body fat.

At some point I came to understand that I was creating the very thing I believed caused me the most pain—excess body fat. In reality, the fat was a byproduct of the pain itself, the pain of not knowing who I was. As I delved deeper into the food, I became less and less connected to myself.

I lived in my body, but it was a stranger to me. I did not know my body at all. Although this separation of the self probably happened early on in my life, each trauma made the split deeper and harder to mend. By the time my son Nicholas died, my body and mind were hanging together like a loose power cord; one trip and the lights would go out.

Right in the middle of this messy life I was making, my husband and I decided it was time to have a baby. My periods were irregular because of PCOS, so it was incredibly challenging to conceive. I joined an online support group for the syndrome and learned that there were several ways of regulating periods with PCOS. One of those ways was low carb dieting. So, I tried "one more time." After doing research for six months on the safest diet, I chose the South Beach Plan, which focuses on limiting healthy carbs and upping protein. It seemed balanced and doable. Six weeks on the plan and I found out I was pregnant. A little over six months into the pregnancy, my son Nicholas was born premature and died a week later.

10

Letting Go

By the time my doctor arrived, my blood had pooled on the hospital room floor. I could hear the nurses' shoes sticking in its thick gooeyness, ripping away from the floor with a loud suck each step they took.

The mad rush to labor and delivery began at 2 am when my placenta erupted from my uterus, sending a thick river of blood down my legs, filling my socks and staining the carpet in our rented house with shades of red. The pregnancy had been complicated from the beginning, but this latest development marked the end at just 28 weeks.

I was very ill throughout the entire pregnancy, from extreme exhaustion to what seemed like the flu. It felt like every bone in my body was broken and floating around inside of me, a gelatinous bag of liquid and fat. It was a bizarre and unsettling sensation, and it propelled my anxiety to new heights. I continued to binge, but somehow I was losing weight. In the first five months, I lost 35 pounds. I felt otherworldly—a stranger in my own body.

A bleeding episode in month six had sent me to the ER, where an ultrasound revealed that I had complete placenta previa. My son's placenta was completely covering my cervix. The bleeding was the result of the placenta tearing away from my uterus. I was sent home and told all would be well.

Just a few weeks later, I nearly bled to death when the placenta tore away entirely. I remember that night clearly. I could not sleep, so, of course, I got up to eat. I put four potatoes on to cook and got out the butter, but before the microwave dinged I was sitting over a blood-filled toilet bowl, shouting for my husband to help me.

Hours later my son Nicholas was born via emergency C-section. I saw him for the first time just after I woke up from anesthesia. He was so small—just one pound and one ounce. Paramedics had to breathe for him with a hand-pumped bag. I knew in my mother's heart he was going to die, even though I was praying as hard as I ever had in my life that he would survive.

I waited in the hall in my hospital bed for the helicopter to arrive to fly him to the nearest children's hospital two hours away. I was physically and emotionally ragged. I felt very much like I wasn't there, like all that had transpired was a Lifetime movie, playing out in some kind of gruesome alternate reality.

After they took him away, they wheeled me back to my room, where I cried well past daylight, stopping only to drink beef broth and to answer calls from Nicholas' pediatrician, who had nothing but dire news for me:

50% chance he will be alive when he gets here,
30% chance he will survive the night,
20% chance he will survive the week,
maybe cystic fibrosis,
maybe intrauterine growth retardation,
maybe,
maybe,

maybe.

Meanwhile, my doctor tried to persuade me to get a blood transfusion, but I refused. It would require a 48-hour hospital stay, and I had to get to the children's hospital to see my son. If I left before I was officially released, my insurance wouldn't pay their part for the birth, so I declined the transfusion and bided my time until my doctor signed me out.

Thirty-six hours after Nicholas was born, my husband and I were on the road to see him. On the way, we stopped for takeout Chinese food, and I binged all the way there. For two hours, I gorged myself on greasy egg rolls, lo mein noodles, and deep friend sweet and sour chicken with extra white rice. I ate and ate and ate. By the time I got there I could no longer feel the pain of my C-section incision or what I knew to be my son's imminent death. I was in a food coma and so sluggish I could barely get out of the car.

Nicholas lived one week in the NICU. I was so blessed to have that time with him, but he went through so much trauma in those seven days that it became clear that letting him go was the most loving thing we could do.

His lungs were not developed, so he was on the last-resort ventilator to keep breathing. He had to have several blood transfusions per day. He had at least six surgeries starting just hours after he was born, and he was on the highest dose of morphine allowed for his little body.

His Dad and I stayed at the Ronald McDonald House across the street from the hospital. We were given access to a kitchen full of free food. Any moment I had away from Nicholas' bed, I ate. I gorged on muffins and donuts and cereal. I filled my plate each evening with the spaghetti and garlic bread made by one of the volunteers. I was so desperate to escape the horror I was living that I would have eaten the world if I could have fit it in my mouth.

In the early morning hours just one week after he was born, we decided to take Nicholas off of life support. I held him outside my body for the first time that night. I looked into his tiny eyes as he took his last breath. When the nurse came to take Nicholas' body from me, I felt as though a hole were ripped in my chest. The hole was deep. It burned and ached, and I knew with a sudden rush of sadness and anger that all the food in the world would not quell that pain. I found myself—again—the mother of a dead child, and from this fact there was no escape. I was broken, body, mind, and soul.

Putting myself back together again would be a task of such enormity that I couldn't fathom it as I stumbled out into the cold daylight that morning. We left the hospital to find our car had two flat tires, and we were down to our last ten dollars. So little of my awareness remained that I crumbled, broken, on the hospital steps. Thanks to the generosity of a stranger, our tires were repaired, and we drove the long two hours home without our son. I feared walking in the door, knowing that the last time I was there my son was still alive; I was still pregnant. I knew I would find the evidence of our trauma everywhere—the blood on the living room carpet, the potatoes rotting in the microwave, my bed piled with clothes and empty suitcases where Nick had rifled quickly through our things to pack a bag for our stay by the children's hospital, but all that could be cleaned up once I regained my strength. The boxes of little clothes and toys waiting for Nicholas in what would have been his room could not. They were haunting me as I watched the sun rise higher in the sky through the brown, leafless tree branches that lined the highway. I had so much joy and hope the day I bought those little sleepers and blankets. Now, I had to somehow ignore the contents of his room until I could decide what to do with those little things. As we walked in the door, I held my breath and then immediately took to the couch, where I would stay until I made myself get up again.

Following Nicholas' memorial service and funeral, I made my way back into the classroom. Spring quarter had just begun, and I was teaching two sections of Women and Writing and taking two graduate courses, like usual. As much as I didn't want to go, I knew that finding my way back to a normal routine would help with the absolutely crippling anxiety that I had developed. It did, but not enough.

Whether it was the trauma of Nicholas' death, my near death or the change of hormones following his sudden birth, I was struggling with the biggest battle of my life—against my own thoughts. I realize now that I was, once again, in the midst of the early stages of post-traumatic stress disorder (PTSD), but then I felt neurotic and out of control. I spent days and days crying and fearing that I would die. I couldn't stand to be left at home alone. And when I was, I ate. I ate and ate and ate. We had so little money that all I could afford was junk food, and I ate it all. I didn't cook. I couldn't cook. I ate Little Debbie's and cheap sweet treats. What I didn't know then was that the sugar was making the anxiety worse. The more of it I ate, the faster my heart would race and the more deranged my thoughts would become. After months of living in some kind of liminal space that seemed far away from any kind of reality I had ever known, I decided to go to the ocean.

After being diagnosed with Polycystic Ovarian Syndrome (PCOS), I made it my mission to know everything I could about the syndrome and to help educate other women as well. I found several support groups online and became an active member on many discussion boards. When I learned that the Polycystic Ovarian Syndrome Association was holding their national conference in New Jersey, I decided I had to go. I needed to connect with other women like me. I needed to be in a room of other women who would understand what it was like to bury a child. I needed to hug other big, beautiful women who were struggling just like me. The added bonus was getting to go to the ocean for the first time in my life. My soul needed the water, but I had no idea how much until my toes hit the sand.

We arrived in Atlantic City just as the sun was coming up. I saw the ocean for the first time from my car window. Its blue expanse stretched out farther than my eyes could see, and I was in awe. We found a place to park near the boardwalk, and I broke into a run, feeling the ocean pull me in. I was both afraid and mesmerized. I quickly stripped off my socks and shoes and rolled up my pants. I held my breath as I stood on the water's edge, allowing the tide to wash swirling waves of cool water over my toes. For the first time since Nicholas died, I felt peace. I sat down in the wet sand and wept long and hard. I felt the deepest, darkest part of my grief ooze into the ocean with each tear.

After breakfast, we changed into our swimsuits and headed out into the water. It was unseasonably warm for early June, but the beach was peppered with only a few other swimmers. I waded in slowly and stood still as the first wave came crashing in, knocking me into the surf. I giggled. I laughed and laughed and laughed. It felt strange, foreign, the sound of my own mirth bubbling out of my body, barely audible above the roar of the water. I released my anger and sadness and guilt right there in the waves and knew for the first time in months that I would be okay. The ocean was so much bigger than me and my problems that it washed away all of my woes. That day, the ocean became my higher power.

I had never been a religious person. My family did not attend church, but I did spend a decent chunk of my childhood sampling other peoples' churches. I went with my friends and neighbors. I felt like I might be missing something. In fact, as my life went on, I would become a member of several different churches. I was baptized in the Church of Christ when I was nine months pregnant with my daughter Samantha. I was confirmed in the Catholic Church not long after my son Nicholas died. But nowhere in any church service or Bible reading or group breakout session did I find the God of my understanding.

But that day on the beach I felt so small, and for the first time in my life I believed that I was part of something larger than my own thoughts. The ocean, so vast and strong, put my own obsession with individuality into perspective. I am my own individual, but I am so much less and so much more. I spent the next decade trying to figure out what happened in those waves.

11

Finding Me

It turns out that the Self cannot easily be forgotten. It was always there, calling my name, waving its hand in hopes of recognition. I will be forever grateful that I finally waved back and escaped my torturous relationship with food that prevented me from truly knowing the most important person in my life: myself.

The search took me in a myriad of directions, from crystals and gems to numerology and astrology. I wandered down many paths in search of my connection to the divine and to myself. Although I never came back empty handed, none of my explorations led to a lasting, satisfying relationship with my higher Self, which is what I was searching for. Finally, I discovered meditation, and I learned not only how to find peace within myself but how to truly love myself in light of being divine.

After an epic, 20-year battle with infertility and learning to cope with the twin tragedies of infant loss and miscarriage, I found out I was pregnant with my only living child, Tristan, during a deep meditation. I had turned to meditation, along with other stress reduction techniques, like massage and deep breathing, in order to increase my chances of getting pregnant, something I had started to think might not ever be possible.

One night toward the end of August I lay on my bed breathing in the exotic scent of lavender incense and quietly clearing my mind of that day's slights. I could feel my mind going deeper into a restive state, and images began to appear, like they always do when I meditate. Within minutes, a clear picture took shape. From what I knew to be a womb, a golden baby's arm appeared. I smiled then broke into a giggle, which ultimately disrupted my meditation, and the little arm disappeared. Although I tried to dispel what I believed to be its meaning, I couldn't get it out of my head. Twenty-four hours later, I took a pregnancy test and found out that I was going to have a baby.

Now, whether it was wishful thinking or a true prophecy really doesn't matter to me, but the power of meditation to take me closer to myself, closer to my true Self, was revealed to me that night, and it became a crucial strategy in my recovery from Binge Eating Disorder.

In the chaos following my son's birth and the early days of breastfeeding and diaper changing, I found myself moving further away from this practice, and my binge eating returned. Instead of finding inner peace through quiet, contemplative meditation, I was searching for it at the bottom of a potato chip bag. Food was my old frenemy. It never said no, it never laughed at me, and it never left me when I needed it most. But it also left me rudderless in waves of confusion and sadness. Meditation showed me that I didn't really know myself at all because I had spent all of my adolescence and adult years in a food-obsessed haze, which I preferred to the pain of reality.

When I started meditating again soon after I entered recovery from Binge Eating Disorder, I discovered Deepak

Chopra. His soothing voice guided me to my true Self as I sat in my old gray chair during my son's naptime. It was the best 15 minutes of my day. The chaos was quieted and I was able to finally connect to the inner me. In that silence, I would see glimpses of what Chopra and other gurus refer to as Source—the being/place/element from whence we originated. It was exciting to me to look beyond societal expectations of me, my expectations of me, and to return to a state of pure divine energy. It was through this practice that I overcame one of my biggest self-limiting fears: dying.

I had been afraid of dying since age eight. I remember the moment I realized I would die very clearly. I was in the backyard of our trailer playing on the swing set. I was swinging so high that the swing set posts were popping up out of the ground with each ascension. Up I would swing, higher and higher and higher, the swing set thumping in and out of the ground. Finally, I got so high up that I could see the trailer roof, newly tarred, and that's when it hit me. I could die. I would die. Someday, I would not exist.

I frantically tried to stop the swing. I had to get off. I had to run. I had to get away. Eventually, as my swing chains twisted and turned, I was able to stop by dragging my feet in the grass. I got off, shaking, and ran. I ran and ran and ran. I had no idea where I was going, but I had to get away from these horrifying thoughts, from this one, startling, unyielding truth: one day, I would not be.

I am not sure if it was the danger of swinging so high that brought on this line of thinking, but it stuck with me, from that moment on the swing until 32 years later, sitting in my old gray chair, when I connected with Source and accepted my divinity. Yes, I would die, but I would live on eternally as stardust. I would become something else—part of a tree, leg of a desk, ear of a squirrel. I would live on, just not as I know myself in this lifetime. It was not that I suddenly believed in reincarnation or that I had some kind of spiritual conversion. Instead, I finally accepted what others had believed for millennia: $e=mc^2$. That is, matter never disappears; it just takes a different form.

With my fear of dying gone, I felt lighter—relieved and content. Ironically, I also felt free to truly live my life. The day I made the realization that I was mortal, I vowed to stay up forever so as not to lose one minute of my life. As an eight year old, I lasted 23 hours before I fell asleep, sitting up in my bed. It scared my mother when she saw me there, sitting up and sleeping. I remember her waking me and checking my pulse. I was alive, but really I was half dead. Shortly after, I developed generalized anxiety disorder, and it would haunt me for the next 30 years.

When people advise me to live like I will die tomorrow, I counter their proclamation. I lived like I would die tomorrow, and it was both exhausting and life wasting. Although many things would contribute to my growing anxiety, the fear of nothingness was powerful and disabling. Without a belief in the afterlife, I was left to face the bleak reality of death as my final act. It was yet another uncontrollable factor in my life that I would eat to suppress. By the time I discovered meditation and the knowledge of materiality, I was more than ready to free myself of that self-limiting belief. Its removal paved the way for true recovery and broke down other ways of thinking that had held me back for many years.

I found that I loved meditating, and I worked hard never to miss a daily session. I longed for more time to practice, but my toddler needed most of my waking hours, which I gladly gave him. As my meditation practice relieved many of my disabling thoughts, I got to know myself better than ever. I started to learn what I liked and how I enjoyed spending my time. I was able to give up doing things that didn't fulfill me. Given that science has shown that meditation can rewire the brain, it makes sense that the practice would improve relaxation, clarity, and sense of self. Eventually, I noticed that meditation was also helping me achieve the one objective I wanted more than anything: the elimination of obsessive thoughts about food.

12

Nursing My Obsession

My nipples bulged purple then red with each suck of the breast pump. I had just nursed my newborn son for his 3am feeding, and I struggled to stay awake long enough to pump a few more ounces for my freezer stash. I was going back to work soon, and I needed to build up enough supply for daycare. It didn't help that my output had been chronically low since the day my son was born. After a difficult, 32-hour labor followed by a C-section, my son was taken to the NICU for eight days.

Although I began pumping just hours after giving birth, my son was allowed nothing by mouth until the fourth day. The optimal nursing environment of close contact and frequent nursing was disrupted, but I did what I could to keep up my supply, including eating.

From the moment we got home from the hospital, I ate. I ate out of fear of losing my son. I ate out of fear of being a brand new mother—again. I ate to cope with the post-surgical pain. I ate to quiet the noiseless rush of anger that was surging between me and my husband.

I had an exceptional excuse: I had to keep up my milk supply. The average nursing mother burns 500 extra calories per day. I had to be sure I got in those calories, so I ate. I ate a lot.

Sports drinks are said to increase milk supply. So, I drank it. I drank it a lot.

Lactation cookies and brownies are said to increase milk supply. So, I made them. I made them a lot.

At one point I monitored my caloric intake and discovered I was taking in nearly 4,000 calories a day. And still, my milk supply remained steady at just under enough to fully nourish my son.

Eventually, I had to supplement with formula, but it only made my body work harder to increase my milk supply.

I added Motilium (Domperidone), a digestive drug whose primary side effect is lactation (even in men). I had to have it made at a compounding pharmacy 30 minutes from my house, and since my insurance wouldn't cover the off label use, I paid $150 out of pocket monthly.

In addition, I took 12 capsules per day of Fenugreek, an herb known to increase milk production. Its only side effect was making me smell like a walking waffle. My entire body reeked of maple syrup. Meanwhile, I was gorging on high calorie foods—stuffing myself painfully all day in the name of, ironically, feeding my son.

In the seemingly endless days and nights that Tristan and I spent together that first summer, I suffered with what appeared from the outside to be a very mild version of post-partum depression (PPD), an illness I sought therapy for around the fifth month of pregnancy. Given my history of child loss and mood disorders, I hoped that seeing a therapist during my pregnancy and for at least six months after would prevent PPD entirely. Thankfully, I truly believed it lessened it, but I will never know for sure because I was numbing my fears and sadness with massive quantities of food—literally weighing down my emotions so that I wouldn't have to deal with them.

But like any problem pushed down too long, those feelings manifested themselves in even more disturbing thoughts and behaviors. Since Tristan's Dad was on the road driving trucks for much of the week, I was left alone to care for a newborn. I was scared of everything. Scared that my son would die in his sleep. Scared that he would fall off the bed and break his neck. Scared that he would get sick in the middle of the night and I wouldn't know what to do.

I barely slept. I was paranoid to the point of hearing and seeing things that were not there. Something unseen was coming after my son. I remember months of nighttime terrors, sitting on my bed, staring at the open door, imagining a specter creeping up the stairs. Then, during the day, the shadows would fade and become embodied. I suffered from a severe anxiety and panic disorder. Heart palpitations thrummed on and on all day long. It felt like a living, breathing sound track to my life.

Because I did not feel sad, I did not tell my therapist about these experiences. I let them go. I felt horrible. Always on edge. Always tired, yet restless. I was so happy to be a mother that I continued trying to shake off the anxiety and ate to find short periods of relief. Meanwhile, the sugar was only making matters worse, to the point that my son and I lost our breastfeeding relationship when he was 21 months old. My heart palpitations and chest pain from acid reflux had become so severe that I had to have a radioactive stress test to rule out heart problems. The radioactive isotope used to gather better images of my heart meant that I had to stop breastfeeding for a minimum of 24 hours. That break led to a fissure in our hard-won breast-feeding relationship, and we never got back to it again. I was proud that we had made it that far when the odds were so clearly stacked against us, but once I was no longer trying to produce milk, my eating didn't decrease. In fact, if anything, it increased. Ultimately, a 3am sugar binge led me to salvation and to the path of recovery.

13

My Body Was Rotting
from the Inside Out

Twenty-eight years of bingeing and dieting had finally caught up to me, and the results were obvious to anyone who came near me.

I stank.

My gastrointestinal track was so diseased that I had constant odorous gas, which made my clothes smell. It was painful and embarrassing.

My feet smelled so badly because of my inability to comfortably bend over and wash them that they reeked through my shoes. People could smell my feet while sitting next to me.

My body was overrun with candida from eating so much sugar and flour, and every crevice smelled like death, including my belly button and other skin folds.

I hurt.

My feet were in so much pain from plantar fasciitis from eating an inflammatory diet that waking up in the morning and walking to the bathroom was sheer agony.

My stomach ached with alternating bouts of diarrhea and constipation.

I had to sleep propped up on five pillows because my acid reflux was so severe that being flat took my breath away–literally.

My migraines were out of control. At 10-12 migraines per month, my quality of life was greatly diminished.

My back burned, and I could not make it through the grocery store without leaning on the cart for support.

I was mentally ill.

My anxiety was so severe that I couldn't sleep without the lights on. I thought I was dying daily, and I went to a myriad of doctors seeking treatment for illnesses from which no one my age should suffer.

I would also sink into periodic pits of despair that drove me to eat more and more and to hate myself.

In addition, I suffered from cystic acne, thin, greasy hair, and bursitis in both hips.

And yet, the urge to keep eating was so powerful that even with all of those symptoms, I continued bingeing. I continued to alternate between starving and overeating. I continued to berate myself. I continued to deny that I was sick, even though I was ill in many ways.

I was just 39 years old when I entered recovery, but my body was disintegrating, and I felt helpless to stop my behavior.

For the first time in my life, I knew I had to seek help or I would die. I chose well being over weight loss. I chose me over societal expectations.

On the night I put down the food, I cried to the universe for help. I did not beg to be thin like I had for decades. I did not wish for a bikini body. I did not long for a svelte silhouette in an evening gown. I petitioned for sanity. I called for freedom from food obsession.

On a hot May night around 3am, I was sitting in my favorite chair in my living room. In my lap was a bowl of freshly made buttercream frosting, which was tinted robins-egg blue. It was my third bowl that night. Nine cups of powdered sugar. Three sticks of butter. The Notebook played quietly on the TV, and every time Noah's heart got broken, I cried for him, but I was really crying for me. A month before, I had reached out to the National Eating Disorders Association (NEDA) help line. After 28 years of suffering, I finally began the early stages of accepting that my life was out of control. I could not stop eating. I was/am a food addict.

As my husband and toddler son slumbered peacefully upstairs, I gorged myself on sugar and fat until I felt sick, until my heart was racing at more than 110 beats per minute, until the food no longer tasted good. Every bite tasted more cloying than the last, and yet I continued to spoon it in. To say I was behaving mindlessly is an understatement. I was well out of my mind before I sat down that night, alone in the flickering TV light, comforting myself for having come to the end of another stressful semester of teaching, another birthday party, another graduation party, another summer course prep, another and another and another.

The movie ended, and I put my licked-clean bowl in the sink, rinsing it carefully to hide the evidence of my binge from my husband. In fact, I took the time to carefully cleanse the entire kitchen as though it were a crime scene. All powdered sugar dust carefully swept up from the counters and floor, the mixer scrubbed to a bright shine and lifted back onto its shelf, and all butter wrappers thrown away inside a paper bag.

I was still crying when I dragged my tired, overwhelmed body upstairs to the shower to wash away the shame of having binged again. I had failed again, I thought. Failed my diet. Failed my doctor. Failed my husband. Failed my son. Failed myself. And for the first time in almost 30 years, I knew that if I did not stop bingeing, I would die from it.

Binge eating was killing me.

As the water ran down my back, I cried more. At one point I got down on my knees in the warm spray and called out for help, pitifully weak at first, but then louder and louder. I turned off the water, dried my body, slipped into my nightgown, and fell into bed, sad, scared, and for the first time, completely and utterly honest with myself. I felt bare and raw and desperate. I fell into a deep sleep from which I woke up hung over from eating so much sugar. But in addition to the bloat, stomach pain, and fatigue, I felt resolved. That morning, I abstained from all trigger foods, including caffeine, alcohol, all processed sugars, all flours, and all processed foods. Abstinence was my first step on my road to recovery.

Giving up those foods wasn't a cure. Abstinence, instead, allowed my body, mind, and soul to get clean. Food addiction, like other addictions, robs the sufferer of her Self. Compulsive eating took me away from me. In fact, on the night that I shoveled spoon after spoon of sugar in my mouth, I had no idea who I was. I think I was more afraid to get to know ME without food than anything else. What if I didn't like that person? What if she wasn't worthy? What if she wasn't good?

That first year I found out that I really do love myself in a thousand different ways. I love myself most when I am doing something to help others. It turns out that without the food my life is fuller than I ever imagined it could be. I was only living a quarter of my life while I was still in the food. A quarter!

That first year was magical in many ways. I had power and control over food for the first time I could remember. I had no problem being around former binge foods. I could make them, touch them, but I had no desire to eat them. For me, those foods had become my torturers. As the wicked step-mother says in Everafter in response to Danielle (aka Cinderella) asking if she had ever loved her, "How could one love a pebble in her shoe?" The same was true for me with hyper-palatable foods.

While there does remain a debate about good foods versus bad foods, and about whether abstinence is helpful or harmful in eating disorder recovery, I can only say that I know what works and doesn't work for me. I made those discoveries through persistence and trial and error. For the first year of my recovery I kept a detailed food journal and logged each of my meals in a calorie counting app. I wanted to know what I was eating and when, but I also wanted to know why. Unlike when I had dieted in the past, keeping track of what I was eating was about curiosity and the destruction of one of the biggest impediments to my healing: denial.

Denial is a pervasive part of most eating disorders, and it manifests itself in many different ways in BED. For me, I was in denial about how much I was eating, how it was harming my body, and how it was impacting my mental state. Observing the way foods affected me was instrumental not only in avoiding those foods, but in avoiding them for life.

My main argument in favor of abstinence is that diet is the top line of defense for most illnesses. For instance, in order to treat my migraines, I had to give up chocolate, alcohol, artificial sweeteners and flavors, and caffeine. It was either stop consuming them or continue suffering with severe, hours-long, body-wide pain. The same would be true if I was diabetic or suffered from celiac disease. Some foods were harming me, so I chose to eliminate them from my diet. I was left with an absolute smorgasbord of delicious, healthy foods. How could I complain or want for anything?

During that first year, I also developed a number of other key strategies for recovery. I regularly listened to Overeater's Anonymous speakers. I joined in on phone and email meetings, and I subscribed to their many e-mail lists. I read recovery literature, and I took inventory and tried to dig as deeply as I could to figure out what events in my past may have contributed to the development or worsening of my eating disorder. Although I had become abstinent, at times I wondered if it was the right or best choice for long-term recovery, and then I read Kay Sheppard's book, Food Addiction: Your Body Knows.

Sheppard's book cemented my innate assumptions about how the body responds to certain foods, like processed flours and sugars, and the need to remove those foods from my life. Her careful use of what was then (1993) very minimal but important scientific studies on food addiction and the brain clarified my own experience, especially with foods that really lit up my brain, like candy bars and mashed potatoes. It was her words that convinced me I was on the right path to recovery, and I decided to stay the course by abstaining from hyper-palatable foods. I cannot express my gratitude to Sheppard enough. I honestly believe that had it not been for her book, my disease might have persuaded me to try moderation again, and I wouldn't be here today, living in more serenity than I have ever known in my life.

I have already discussed the powerful role meditation has played in my recovery, and I use other tools to gain centeredness and peace of mind as well. I say the "Serenity Prayer" as often as I repeat the Hindu God Ganesha's mantra to hear my concerns and destroy those obstacles that beset me: "Om gam ganapatye namaha." I create vision boards, not for weight loss hopes as I had in the past, but to help discover my inner Self. I use essential oils for relaxation. I take hot baths late at night after the house is quiet. I draw and color pictures to focus on something outside of myself, and I make beautiful recovery jewelry and other items for my Etsy shop.

Of course, writing has been, and will always be, crucial to anything difficult I face in life. Without writing, I am pretty sure I would have committed suicide as a teenager. Writing gave me an outlet for expression and a place to think and to resolve problems. And as my writing skills improved, it served as a site for rising self-esteem. I started writing this book just months into recovery and started my blog, OptimisticFoodAddict.com, about a year later. Knowing that my words can help others in recovery is a further incentive to keep on writing.

I felt it very important in the first year to keep track of what and how much I was eating, not to punish or restrict myself, but to really look honestly at what I was putting in my mouth. I was able to resolve many of the illnesses that had plagued me from eating too much, especially too much sugar. Within the first six months, my severe, chronic migraines had been reduced to one per month (down from 10-12 per month). In addition, I healed my painful plantar fasciitis, restored my periods, resolved the worst of my anxiety and depression, eliminated my severe rosacea, and just generally felt better. I no longer smelled. I no longer felt unable to care for myself. I felt good.

During that time, I lost 70 pounds. I was proud of my weight loss, but I soon found that I had deep, unresolved issues with my body, my sexuality, and my weight loss. I was feeling more and more at home in my body and found fewer reasons to reach out to food for comfort, but I needed more support. My local Overeater's Anonymous meetings were held at times that were impossible for me to get to without advanced arrangement, so I joined their online groups, which were very helpful to me. Daily e-mails and regular sharing of recovery stories helped me feel less alone. I joined several binge eating support groups on Facebook, and they were helpful in that I was able to see that my relationship with food was disordered but far from unique. However, I quickly learned that the addiction model for treating Binge Eating Disorder was not accepted in any of those groups. Abstinence from trigger foods, like flour and sugar, was frowned upon. Instead, all of the groups to which I regularly posted embraced intuitive eating, which required followers to listen to their bodies and eat what they wanted. Nothing was forbidden. I had tried that approach a few years before, thinking that it would help me better understand my hunger signals. What I found was that it gave me a license to binge, and binge I did.

Although I truly understood and believed in the potential for intuitive eating to be beneficial and healing for some (and still do), it was not the right path for me. Further, the increasing hostility toward my recovery plan, which involved many of the same tools, such as mindfulness, awareness, and getting to know your body, was becoming counterproductive to my well being. Eventually, I struck out on my own and went on to found what has become my lifeline, the Food Addiction Recovery support group on Facebook. The story of that group is my story and our story. It demonstrates the power that strangers with keyboards can have in our lives and in our recovery.

14

A Place of Our Own

After the third debate of the week turned to ugly name calling, I decided to leave the Binge Eating Disorder Facebook group of which I had been a member since the early days of my recovery. It was an incredibly difficult decision because I felt that I was cutting my only lifeline with people who understood what if it was like to gorge myself to the point of physical pain and to beat myself up mentally for days after. At the same time, I knew if I didn't go, I could compromise my recovery and the recovery of others.

The main disagreement centered on supposedly conflicting beliefs about the function of and treatment for BED. There are two main ways that lay people understand compulsive overeating: (1) the intuitive eating model and (2) the addiction model. While this binary is surely overly simplistic, it provides a way of getting at the chaos sufferers face when seeking help for BED.

All of the BED support groups I found on Facebook were formed under the premise that BED was best treated though intuitive eating (IE), a model popularized by Geneen Roth. IE requires followers to not restrict any food or food groups and to see all foods without value or bias. In other words, according to IE, there are no good or bad foods. It is all just food. In addition, followers of this recovery method are urged to be mindful while eating and to eat without distraction—no loud music, no TV, no books, and so on. IE also recommends using a hunger chart to rate hunger levels. All of these tools (and others) are designed to help the binge eater get in touch with his or her own hunger signals and to be able to develop a healthy relationship with food and his or her own body.

While I believe fully in being more mindful about eating and in repairing the mind/body split, I found myself much more in line with the addiction model of recovery. Understanding BED as food addiction means that the binge eater has a physiological reaction to certain foods. Recovery, then, requires abstinence from foods that are likely to cause such a reaction in the brain. Most commonly, these foods contain high levels of sugar, salt, fat, and/or flour, but each individual person in recovery makes his or her own list to determine which foods spike obsessive thoughts about eating. In addition to abstinence, food addicts in recovery practice many of the techniques used in IE, such as mindful eating and listening to the body. The main difference is that IE disallows abstinence. The addiction model of recovery from BED was developed in the 1960s by Rozanne S., who modeled Overeater's Anonymous (OA) after Alcoholics Anonymous (AA). Since then, other groups have taken up OA's original plan and formed their own support programs with abstinence as one of the cornerstones.

From what I can tell from my regular interactions with BED sufferers, neither one of these approaches is more right or more wrong. Given that our scientific knowledge of BED is still in its infancy, it is too soon to speculate on which method of recovery is better than the other. In fact, at some point, a totally different method of treatment might be developed. Recently, several new drugs have been released for the treatment of BED, but, again, the science is new and far from conclusive.

Nonetheless, after trying and failing with IE, I committed to abstinence and found sustained serenity there for the first time in nearly 30 years. Unfortunately, every time I tried to share my experiences with others in various BED Facebook groups, my comments were hotly debated and often erased by moderators. At first I was angry. I felt like I was being silenced, just like I had been my entire life, but eventually I realized that the moderators had a right to what they believed to be the best, most helpful path of recovery, so I dropped out of all of the BED groups I was in and formed my own group called Food Addiction Recovery (FAR). Within days, the group had swelled to 300 members. As of this writing, we are 6,425 members strong.

In the early days of the group, I felt it was important to allow it to grow organically. What did our members need in order to recover well? How could our Facebook group become and remain a safe place for people in recovery from BED? Although there have been squabbles from time to time over what is allowed to be posted, the FAR group has been an overwhelmingly positive and safe place to share recovery strategies and get support. Unlike many other Facebook groups in which I have been a member, the FAR group has rarely been a site for personal attacks or hateful responses. In fact, I have been surprised by the open, caring, generous support given so freely among these strangers with keyboards.

As we grew, our membership rules changed and were shaped largely from the experiences of group members and literature written about BED recovery. Our strongest point, though, is that the group recognizes and appreciates the addiction model of recovery, while accepting that other means of recovery can also be viable. Within that flexible framework, some rigidity was required for what I believe to be the best interests of our members:

No diet talk, because our group is not a weight loss group. Given that many BED sufferers first developed their eating disorders from dieting and weight loss efforts, we desperately needed a place that was free from weight loss and diet methods.

No before and after photos. The primary reason behind this restriction is that those photos can trigger people into wanting to diet, which can trigger people into binge-ing. But another reason why before and after photos are not allowed to be posted in the group is because they are a remnant of diet culture. They represent dissatisfaction with an older, fatter body, which is really dissatisfaction with the self.

No selling of dieting products or any other materials or services. It became obvious early on that we had to be mindful of people who saw us as sitting ducks, a captive marketplace. Since BED sufferers are often susceptible to quick fixes and magic bullets, making a steadfast rule about selling anything of any kind made the most sense.

No food pictures or recipes. Pictures of food and directions on how to prepare food can trigger people with BED, so it is simpler to ban them than to take a chance on someone lapsing or relapsing.

But the No's are not what makes the group work so well. It is the many, many Yes's that make it my favorite place in cyberspace. I have seen so much wonderful compassion in the group that I have been moved to tears on many occasions. In addition, true, loving relationships have developed among members, including me. At around the end of the second year of its existence, I reached out to two members who were especially devoted to the group to help me moderate, and it made a world of difference. Not only did it allow me to focus more on my own recovery, but I was able to start building more means of support for our members through my website OptimisticFoodAddict. com. The website features my blog, helpful guides on recovery for beginners, and other resources for people with BED. I was also able to create a free writing course and a therapeutic coloring book. All of these tools have been created to serve as recovery lifelines and to augment other recovery strategies.

Our members use many tools in their recovery, including meditation, mindful eating, Overeaters Anonymous attendance, both online and in person, Food Addicts Anonymous, Celebrate Recovery, pharmaceutical options, abstinence, writing, art therapy, exercise, gratitude, and on and on. I found that by leaving the doors and windows open to as many healthy routes to recovery as possible, our members have been able to find peace from obsessive thoughts and behaviors around food. There may never be one way to recover from BED, and the diversity of our members' strategies demonstrates that that is more than okay. As much as we are on our own individual paths of recovery, we have found that we do far better when meeting up along the way than we do when keeping our heads down. Regrettably, it took many years for me to understand that I could not do this alone and many more to even accept that I suffered from an eating disorder.

CHRISTINA FISANICK GREER

15

Loving the Fat Girl

As old-timers tell us, the first year is about what not to do. The second year is about what you do. At the end of the first year, I felt great, empowered, in touch with ME, and capable of making great decisions. Then, something happened in the second year that made me realize that recovery, for everyone, has its ebbs and flows.

After going back to campus in the fall semester, dozens of colleagues and students kept complimenting me on my weight loss. At this point, I had lost 75 pounds. At first I was flattered, but then, it began grating on me.

People were staring at me.

Why were they looking at me?

Why were they noticing my body?

Stop it.

Stop it, okay?

These negative emotions hit their zenith at the end of the first week of classes when I walked into my neighborhood coffee shop for a piece of fruit and some tea. As soon as I opened the door, I wanted to run and hide. A table full of men at least 15 years my senior stopped talking and stared at me as I walked through the small shop. They leered at me. I could feel their eyes scanning my breasts, my hips, and my ass. Suddenly, I was 11 years old again. I felt like I was being devoured, violated, and abused.

I got my tea and walked slowly to my car.

I cried the entire hour to work.

I did not binge that day. I did not binge the next day, but slowly my portion sizes began to creep up. They got a little bigger at each meal. I stopped keeping track of what I was eating. I slowly stopped meditating. Before I knew it, I was on the slippery slope and heading for a binge. I tried over and over again to re-right myself, but it would last only a week or so before I was slipping into larger portions again.

Thankfully, I maintained my abstinence from trigger foods. If not for that, I am certain I would have started bingeing again. But I KNEW that if I did, I might not come back from that dark and desperate place. I wrote about what I was feeling. My therapist and I processed my childhood experiences with sexual violation, and little by little, I regained my foothold over this disease.

I never let go of my recovery. I just loosened my grip.

What did I learn in year two?

No one has perfect recovery. No one.

Starting over every time I slip up is left over from diet mentality.

Starting over does not offer me a new beginning but an excuse to wallow in my addiction.

Abstinence is essential to making good decisions in recovery and in life.

Being in recovery is not the same as living in recovery.

I will be living in recovery for the rest of my life.

I need to stay in close contact with my inner self. Once that connection weakens, it gets harder to re-strengthen.

Gratitude is essential to my recovery.

Giving back to others is essential to my recovery.

Being honest with myself and about myself is essential to my recovery.

A recovery plan that works for me today may not work for me tomorrow.

Just moments ago I started crying, not from sorrow but from disbelief, from joy, from gratitude, from serenity. I have been humbled by this second year. I have been stripped of my EGO. In its place is a wholeness of a kind I never knew before recovery. I like myself. I like being around myself. I like spending time with myself. I no longer feel the need to hide from my feelings and fears. If they come, I let them wash over me, knowing that they will go as they came.

As for the men in the coffee shop, I saw them again several months later. I smiled at them, disarming them far more than a sneer ever could. I can't say that I am healed in regards to sexual abuse, but I can say that I am stronger than I have ever been before.

I knew, after all of that, that there would be rough days in my recovery ahead. Since I live in my recovery, it would necessarily be complicated. I also knew that I now had a toolset to face and possibly prevent relapse, but decided to live in the now as much as I could. By staying in the moment, I had a better chance of maintaining my serenity. But life is messy, and sometimes the only option we have in the end is to clean it up.

CHRISTINA FISANICK GREER

16

Washing Away

"Use the vanilla one, Mama," instructed my three year old son as he watched me test the water temperature for our bath.

"This one?" I asked, holding up a purple bottle of Calgon lavender and vanilla. We had just gone shopping for new "bubble stuff" that afternoon and he was excited to try it.

"Yeah!" he shouted, struggling to slip off his tie-dyed t-shirt and jean shorts.

He watched as I poured a capful into the warm running water. "Look at all those bubbles!"

I put the cap back on the bottle and slipped out of my nightgown. I stepped into the fragrant water and held my hands out for him to join me. Bubble baths had become our weekly ritual, and we both looked forward to the quiet, and sometimes not-so-quiet, merriment in the bubbles.

After taking our seats, we talked about what we did on the playground earlier that day and how glad we were to be outside for the first time in a couple of days. August had started off rainy and cool, and we had finally hit a hot day.

He said he'd really enjoyed the slide, and before I knew it, he was acting out his new maneuvers by sliding down my soap-slippery thigh, which I had propped up to make room in the bubbles for both of us.

On what seemed like the fiftieth trip from my knee to my groin, he said he was tired.

"I'm just gonna snuggle on your tummy, Mama," he told me, wrapping his arms around my white, expansive flesh. He put his head down and whispered, "So comfy and cozy."

I looked at him there, resting peacefully on my belly, and saw my body in a completely different light. What had been a saggy, stretch-marked blob to me moments before had become a luxurious pillow cradling my son's head. I immediately realized that I could no longer loathe this part of my body. Not only had it grown a new life, but it was now giving that life pleasure and comfort.

Just months before, I had started taking pictures of myself in the tub to measure my weight loss progress. As more of the tub sides appeared, I became more gratified that my recovery plan was working, but what I didn't realize was that with each click of my camera phone, I was undoing my own best efforts. Although research on binge eating disorder is still in its infancy, it has become clear that dieting and weighing in are counterproductive to recovery from the disorder.

Despite knowing that calorie counting would likely keep me in the binge-restrict cycle, I felt that I had to keep track of my caloric intake in order to be accountable. Many BED therapists recommend keeping a food journal for this reason, but calorie counting is often discouraged because it lends itself to further food obsession and further distance from the body.

I quickly came to see that before and after photos were harmful in many ways. While they motivate people to go on diets, and maybe even stick to them for a while, the motivation doesn't last long, partly because it comes from a place of body hatred and disgust. It is hard to make permanent changes that are based on self-loathing. If I wanted to recover from binge eating disorder, weight loss had to be a side effect. It could not be the goal. I had spent my whole life chasing a bikini body, and I realized for the first time that it wasn't mine. The body I wanted was someone else's. In fact, it was imaginary. It was make believe me.

Early one morning I woke up warm in my bed. I was curled up into a fetal position, and I slowly slid the covers off and let my hand glide down my side and rest for a moment in the space between my ribs and hip. It felt good sitting in that soft spot. I opened my eyes to look down and see what my hand was feeling and was shocked.

That's not what I am supposed to look like!

Instead of falling into an immediate bad mood, I stopped myself. What exactly did I mean? How was I supposed to look? According to whom?

I realized that the image of the perfect female body had been literally imprinted on my brain over years and years and years of seeing that image and being told that it was RIGHT. When I looked down at my own living, changing body, I expected to see a model's body. It was instant cognitive dissonance.

And I was angry!

My own body, which I had just adored and caressed lovingly, had become a defected, not-enough thing in under a second.

I remember an art teacher telling me once that I would never be an artist because I did not draw what I saw, but I drew what I remembered. This was true in that moment, and probably had been true for decades. I was not really seeing my body as it was. Instead, I was looking at my body through society's lens, and I couldn't be angrier.

I scrambled out of bed and stood before the mirror on the back of my closet door. There, right there, I was. Since my art teacher was right and I could not draw well, I traced my body with pink lipstick right on the mirror. I marveled at the dips and rises of my thighs. I lingered in the space between my neck and clavicle. I giggled as I rounded my hips.

When I was done outlining my form, I stood back and marveled at my work. This outline in pink was MY body shape. It was not Photoshopped. It was not perfect. It was the shape of a 39-year old woman who had given birth to three children, had had her gallbladder and tonsils removed, and who loved to swim, loved to ride her bike, and loved to dance in the kitchen with her tabby cat on Friday nights.

I fell to my knees and cried, calling out until I went hoarse:

I love you!

I love you!

I love you!

I meant it. I did not need to be a size two, a size eight, a size 16, or a size 20 to love my body. I did not need validation from anyone outside myself to love my body. Right at that moment, I loved my body more than I had in decades. That pink outline, drawn crudely in the early morning light, made my body visible to me again.

Eventually, I got up off of the floor, washed the mirror, and took a shower. I felt whole, clean, and new, riding the wave of that beautiful morning well into the rest of the week.

17

Hugging

The day after they buried their mother, we met for dinner; childhood friends I hadn't spent any kind of real time with in more than 25 years. More than 20 people came to the local Italian restaurant where my friends' mother and father had dined on their honeymoon. Much like the funeral, there was much laughter and sharing of stories from days gone by.

Their house was in the middle of a trailer court. Five trailers flanked each side of their white house and wide yard. Our landlord had tried for years to buy their house and yard, but the Halls stuck with the house that their ancestors had built, and I am glad they did. I was closer to them than I was my own cousins, and it was never clearer to me how much we loved each other than on that bitter cold night in January.

I was 19 months into my recovery then, and reaching ever toward the end of my second year. The prior seven months had been a rollercoaster, unlike the high of the majority of my first year. I had relapsed three times—not on foods that I knew I needed to avoid, but first on green tea lattes, then on dried corn, then on portions in general. The last one was the hardest to battle.

I had promised myself at the outset that I would stop calorie counting at the end of my first year of recovery. I hit my one-year anniversary and deleted the calorie-tracking app from my cell phone. I could feel myself edging toward food and weight obsession again. It was starting to worry me.

As we sat around the table reminiscing about our childhood days and catching up on the years in between, the time came to order, and the only abstinent item on the menu was a small tossed salad with vinegar and oil. As my friends enjoyed the restaurant's signature homemade pasta and sauce, I ate my tiny meal and listened.

One of the blessings of not being food obsessed is being able to be fully present. Just two years before, my mind would have been on the food.

Will two meatballs be enough?

If I eat this entire plate, will they think I'm a pig?

I hope no one eats the last slice of bread.

I really shouldn't eat so much butter.

All the while, I would have missed the news of the recent baby being born, Gina going to nursing school, and Donnie's break up. I want to be present—I need to be present—for those kinds of moments. They were why I was there in the first place. Being present requires nothing more than being content in the moment.

After the plates were taken away and the check was settled, Theresa asked how I liked the spaghetti. I told her I had a salad instead. She objected loudly, "You can't come to the best pasta place in the Valley and eat a bowl of lettuce!"

I leaned in, brushing the hair out of my eyes, and explained, "You know how some people are addicted to drugs or alcohol? Well, I am in recovery for food addiction."

"So, you sat there and watched us eat all this food?" she asked, obviously dismayed.

"Sure, but it didn't bother me. It hasn't bothered me in a long time. Foods like that take me away from all of you, and myself."

It felt good to explain it so clearly, even if she might not have truly understood what I meant.

"Well, that's great!" she said with the same kind of fervor as her earlier dismay.

Soon, we were all putting on our coats and heading outside for a picture. We needed a snapshot, a still image, a digital record to commemorate the occasion. As our server struggled with our Smartphones on the dimly-lit sidewalk, I found myself bubbling inside. Happy. At peace. Content. For the fist time in years, I felt like I belonged. These people knew me. They knew all my wars and faults. They knew I could be selfish and vain and dogmatic and judgmental. And yet, they still loved me. They still wanted me to say farewell to their mother and to share in their sorrow and joy. Most of all, they still wanted to embrace me—really.

When we were certain that we got one good shot, our crowd began to disperse under a hail of hugs. I eagerly wrapped my arms around them, sometimes two of them at a time, but it wasn't until I finally hugged Theresa that I realized just how wonderful it felt to be held by someone who loves me. And I knew then that this was a recovery breakthrough. A major recovery breakthrough. And it was a sign that something fundamental had shifted in me, deep in my marrow. After all, I had avoided hugs and most other kinds of physical contact with others since early childhood.

I never felt I was good enough. I was also worried about how my body would feel or smell to the other person. But through the process of recovery, I not only learned how to appreciate my own body, but to finally let others appreciate it as well. Hugs had never felt so wonderful.

18

Dancing with the Dragon

The fever started the day after Christmas, and by December 28, I was out of commission entirely—struck down by the flu. I could barely sleep, but that's all I wanted to do. My throat hurt, my head hurt, my back hurt. My entire body was alive with peculiar aches and painful spasms.

By the time I started feeling somewhat functional, I still had no appetite and, worse yet, no sense of smell or taste. This predicament gave me a good opportunity to put to rest a curiosity that had plagued me for decades: what role does taste and smell play in bingeing?

We know from recent research and self-admissions that companies engineer foods that make it impossible "to eat just one." Given the purposeful nature of hyper-palatable foods to make us crave more and more, what happens when taste and smell are no longer in play? Of course, our sensory experience of food involves texture, visual appearance, and even sound (recall the crunch of a pretzel or the snap of a Slim Jim), but most food addicts I know have immediate reactions to trigger foods once they hit their tongues.

There's a saying in recovery circles: Alcoholics and drug addicts keep their dragons (addictive substances) in cages, while food addicts walk their dragons three times per day. Well, for the sake of my one burning question, and at the risk of derailing my recovery, I decided to dance with the dragon.

I planned my experiment for New Year's Eve. Still not hungry from being ill, I chose my mother's Christmas cookies as my test. They were rich butter cookies piled high with too-sweet cream cheese frosting. My mother made these cookies for the first time that year, so I did not have a nostalgic relationship with them as I do with some of my trigger foods, like mashed potatoes, pancakes, and bananas.

To begin my experiment, I placed two cookies on a plate. They were heart-shaped and decorated with stiff, white icing. I sniffed them. I could smell nothing. I sat down in my chair to finishing watching It's a Wonderful Life for the fifth time that season, and I took a small bite of the first cookie. It had absolutely no flavor. The shock of the cookies that I had expected never came, but given I hadn't eaten that much that day, or really for much of the week, I figured I would finish both cookies and go off to bed.

But that's not what happened. Despite the fact that the cookies had no flavor whatsoever, I ended up going back into the kitchen again and again, eating six cookies total. Once her cookies were gone, I ate a sleeve of Oreos. Although my stomach physically hurt from eating too much, an hour after my experiment began, I found myself standing in front of the microwave waiting for three slices of my homemade lasagna to heat. I was in full-on binge mode.

I woke up the next morning hungry, but not ravenous. I gave myself permission to eat whatever I liked, but I chose to eat healthy, abstinent foods. My senses of taste and smell had mostly returned, but I just wanted miso soup instead of noodle soup and grapefruit over Hershey's kisses.

I was bewildered, and even more so once I made my way to the grocery store for the fist time in days. Once there, I gave myself direct, unimpeachable permission to buy whatever I wanted, including my most favorite of all binge foods—two chocolate cookie sandwiches with butter cream frosting in the middle. I must have eaten those cookie sandwiches a dozen times right in my car. I could never get out of the parking lot without gobbling them both down. As I passed the bakery case I could smell the cakes and breads baking, and to my great surprise, instead of feeling tempted, I felt repulsed. I spotted my former go-to-binge food and felt sick. As I tried to recall the way they tasted, I shuddered like I had swallowed something revolting and walked on.

Not long ago, I would have been kicking myself over not taking the opportunity to eat those cookie sandwiches, but at this point, I have no attachment to that decision. For once, the cookies have become what they are—cookies.

Of course, I don't recommend that anyone with an eating disorder attempt such an experiment. My therapist was both genuinely curious and sincerely annoyed at the risk I took that night, but I'm glad I did it. Now I know that taste and smell are not the only binge triggers. Clearly something happens in my brain when I ingest sugars and flours.

19

Lapse. Relapse. Near Collapse. Or, Green Tea Lattes and the Law of Diminishing Returns

The barista slid the 16 ounce iced, green frothiness over the pick-up counter, and I smiled at it with eager anticipation, and maybe even a bit of trepidation. I had read about green tea lattes on a Facebook page I follow, and I decided to try one. Given that the recommender was a health coach who specialized in Polycystic Ovarian Syndrome, I didn't question the drink's healthfulness, but I should have.

As I strolled through the department store with my toddler, sipping the green tea latte goodness, I was continuously surprised by the flavor of what I thought was a low sugar drink. Little did I know that long before my straw ever found the last tasty slurps, I would be hooked, and the battle to give up the cold drink would eventually lead to a relapse.

Two hours after I first placed my order, I realized that I was high on sugar and caffeine for the first time in more than 14 months. By 2 a.m., long after my son was already asleep and my husband had left for work, I found myself deep in the process of decluttering my entire first floor.

Hours later, I lay awake, unable to sleep and full of ideas for writing projects, the house, and my life. Finally, I tracked down the information on the green tea latte and was startled to find that, when made with soy milk, it contained more sugar than anyone should ingest. I hadn't had that much sugar, or any caffeine, in well over a year, and I was shocked by the effect. Unfortunately, neither caused the usual heart palpitations and anxiety, so I deluded myself into believing that I'd found my latest Starbucks drink, without the added syrup, of course.

Soon, I had upgraded from a grande to a venti to a trenta. I was driving to Starbucks twice a day to get my fix, which sometimes meant driving half an hour to make it to the only Starbucks that was open late. Within a week, I found myself spending upwards of $15 a day, not including gas money, on green matcha lattes. Yes, I realized that I was quickly becoming obsessed and quite possibly excessive. To lower the burden, I ordered the mix so that I could make them from home. I used both boxes within three days.

Each morning I would wake up tired, unmotivated, and yearning for my green drink.

My decluttering project, which had begun as a gentle entrée into minimalism, became an obsessive fling fest fueled by sugar and caffeine. I found myself staying up well into the morning hours, throwing away and boxing up things I no longer wanted—clothes that were now too big, an extra punch bowl, tea serving sets, serving trays, cloth dinner napkins, never-read books, wall hangings, worn-out shoes. Day after day I'd load up my car with boxes for donation and my trash cans with junk. While each night, with little regard for the online classes I was teaching or any part of the rest of my life, I chanted with my three year old: "Keep or donate?" "Keep or donate?" until I had rooted out all excess hiding behind closed doors in my finished basement and first floor.

Since I was using green matcha lattes as meal replacements, my weight started dropping after a long stall, and I proclaimed outwardly that the drinks gave me the boost I needed to get the work done. I refused to employ my own recovery tools: self-love, abstinence, gratitude, and honesty.

And I relapsed.

The mindless eating crept in like a thief, the way it always has before. An extra piece of tofu here. A larger slice of watermelon there. Until I found myself standing in the kitchen after dinner eating natural peanut butter with a knife because I had already used all of the clean spoons. The next night I ate a giant bowl of air-popped popcorn smothered in oil and salt while I read, of all things, a book on abstinence.

I was in trouble. I kept telling myself that I wasn't bingeing, but I wondered nervously how many bites away I was. I was eating recklessly, mindlessly. And I knew that the first step to regaining mastery was to let go.

Two weeks later I stopped drinking green matcha lattes. It wasn't "just like that," but it was cold turkey.

I owe some of this change to my husband.

Sitting in the kitchen one morning, he asked me what was on my mind. I thought for a few minutes, and then carefully explained.

"I wake up in the morning and begin planning my day around when I will get my green tea latte. And I spend the evening rushing through activities so I can make it to Starbucks on time. I know this isn't right, but how wrong is it?"

"That does sound pretty extreme," he replied, sipping on his own coffee shop concoction.

He said nothing for a few minutes and then added, "But it could be worse. At least you're not in fear of losing your job because of it." He's usually good at looking at the whole picture.

"I guess so," I argued against my own case, "but counting gas, I am spending nearly $20 a day on drinks."

He paused, then said, "Well, you have to ask yourself if it is worth getting into an accident with our son in the car. I mean, I see it every day on the same road you drive on."

We both got quiet, and I started loading the dishwasher. By the time I pressed the "start" button, I had made a decision, which I announced shortly after I heard the water come on. "I'm giving it up tomorrow."

"There's no need for that," my husband countered, thinking he might have made too harsh an argument.

"No, it's time," I assured him as I picked up a rag and started wiping down the counter tops.

"What if you switched to once a week? Why not moderation?" he asked, getting up from the table and walking toward the living room.

"Clearly, one drink is too much and never enough," I said as I picked up a basket of folded laundry and headed up the stairs to my son's room. I paused in his doorway, basket in hand, and watched his abdomen rise and fall in the morning light that was seeping through the window blinds.

After putting away the laundry, I went down the steps and out to the car, where I had left last night's latte cup. I picked it up, walked to the outdoor trash cans, ready for morning pick up, and tossed it in.

Reflecting on what happened during this one month green tea latte spree helps provide clues to understanding how food addiction functions, at least for me.

On the day I took my first sip, I got high. There is no doubt about it. Within hours I was exuberant, energized, and for lack of a more precise word, buzzed. I felt like I had before I stopped bingeing. Back then it took way more sugar to achieve that feeling of elation, but my year-long abstinence must have re-set my threshold.

Each time thereafter, when I rushed to order a green tea latte, I was looking to experience that same euphoria. In fact, I was desperately seeking that ur or uber high, the original high, the first time I had left my body and pain and situation through food. I was trying to escape reality with each sip.

Regrettably, or maybe fortunately, the Law of Diminishing Returns, which is as true and fundamental to me as the Law of Gravity, proves that each bite, drink, or snort after the first exalting one can never yield that same response.

While it was happening, I knew what I was doing. Unlike in the past when I would have ferociously defended my poor choices, my attempts to do so this time were weak and easy to dismantle:

It's my only vice.

It can't be that bad.

It's healthy, though.

I can use it as a meal replacement.

I am not hungry when I drink it.

All of those things are true on some level, but I knew that my green tea latte drinking days were numbered. So, I quit.

This experience reinforced my knowledge that one of the major components of my version of BED is food addiction. I am a sugar addict. I am a caffeine addict. I am an addict. One bite is one too many, yet it can never be enough.

It also reminded me, yet again, that nothing lasts forever. One bite DOES mean that I'm in for a hell of a ride, but it doesn't mean I can't get back off. I fully acknowledge that I will live with this disease for the rest of my life, but I also believe, for the first time ever, that I am not doomed to failure. It will not best me.

I have no intention of tempting fate and risking my well being, but I also know that this will not be the last time I encounter a substance, a person, an event, or a thing that triggers my addiction. With the three recovery mantras: self-love, honesty, and gratitude, I believe I will be capable of finding my way back to sanity should this ever happen again.

Now that I have lived free from the influence of addictive foods for so long, I know it is worth every effort to regain and maintain my recovery. I believe that serenity is my natural state. Anything else is insanity.

20

I Stand Here Scraping

"I stand here ironing, and what you asked me moves tormented back and forth with the iron." -Tillie Olsen

On the fourth day, they painted the window frames gold, and that's when I fired them.

It took us all summer to hire an exterior painting crew. Few painters returned our calls and the ones who did either refused to do the job we expected, or offered us bids that were double their competitors. We decided on A-One Painting more out of haste from the quickly fading summer than because we believed they'd do the best job.

After nearly two weeks of no shows, mistaken paint colors, and half-assed scraping, the owner returned my money less the minimal work already completed. This left us little choice other than to paint the house ourselves.

At the outset it seemed entirely doable. My husband and I, along with our family and friends, set out with rollers and ladders to conquer our 1926, two-story stucco house. As the days wore on, however, it became obvious that this was a bigger job than anyone anticipated. Every evening after work I found myself scraping, peeling away at the decades of hardened paint until near sunset.

Soon, I began to look forward to this ritual. The rhythmic movement of scraping soothed me, but more so, the uncovering of the original stucco, inch by inch, had me hooked. Layer upon layer of old paint yielded to my blade as I etched deeper into the thick coating, down past cream to green to blue to what I think might have been yellow, all the way down to the original stucco. Clean. Both smooth and rough. It was as if I was reclaiming the house as my own. Removing all of the years of others' choice and work to find the house's core, as it was before anyone decided to change it to suit their style.

By the fifth night, I came to see how my recovery was much like my house's rehab. Recovering from food addiction, for me, is about getting to my true Self, figuring out what my inner me is like, without the imposition of others and without seeing myself through what I imagine their lenses for seeing me might be.

As the weeks went by, the methodical scrape, scrape, scraping was wired into my day as much as my meditation ritual. The rhythm of my arm, hand, and scraper allowed me to think. I worked alone on my side of the house. At first I thought it was too quiet, and the drumbeat of that day's woes played on in my mind as paint chips flew onto my hair, clothes, and shoes. But soon, I became mindful of the world around me. The sun was warm on my back. It deflected the chill of the breeze, which was strong enough to blow paint dust into my mouth, despite the mask I donned. My goggles were comfortable on my face, but the right lens had fogged, obscuring my peripheral vision. As my gloved right hand worked on a stubborn hump of dried paint, I heard bird song coming from the pine tree in our front yard. Our mourning doves had long since left their nest beneath our porch eaves, and we missed their song. I dug on, grateful to see a large patch of original stucco starting to appear, its grainy, gray surface now exposed to the light and wind for the first time in decades.

Each day I scraped a little more, getting lost in my work. I focused on myself and the old paint for those hours in the fading, autumn sun, so grateful for the time to contemplate.

Soon, it became obvious that the job was too big for us to handle alone; the house was too big to be scraped. So, we hired an experienced painter to help us apply new stucco and to paint the soffit and fascia. He came highly recommended by our good friend, who was an indoor painter. We had met him before, and he seemed knowledgeable about his trade.

The day Frankie arrived we put him to work right away on the stucco. His long hair was tied up in a ponytail, and his wife beater revealed an interesting mix of tattoos here and there. I was amazed by his strength. Stucco mixes are heavy, and yet he lifted the container of gray mud to his platform like it was a basket of greens from the garden. I watched as he troweled on the thick mix, first coating the side of the house with a thick layer, then using another trowel to add uniformity and texture. I missed scraping. I missed the hours working in the lingering sunlight, but I yielded to my husband and Frankie. After all, the house needed painting, and the time remaining to do so before winter made it impossible to keep going.

After a week of hard work, Frankie had managed to cover half of one side of our house in stucco. It looked good. Smooth and cool, light gray amidst the sage grass. Frankie's labors made it possible for Jim and me to concentrate on prepping the window frames for painting. One Saturday morning, as the three of us labored on, Jim accidentally hit the new stucco with his scraper handle and a chunk of the cement fell off. We looked at each other with a dawning sickness. I held my breath as he pushed the blade into the newly-formed opening, and nearly wept as a sheet of grey stucco as big as my hand flaked off and fell to the ground, shattering into dozens of crusty pieces and sending a gray cloud of dust onto his feet. Within seconds, we had both peeled off an entire wall of the cement laid just days before by Frankie.

Jim threw his scraper down into the grimy heap and began pacing as I had seen him do many times over the years. He was furious. I wondered what he would say to Frankie, who, having seen what happened to his work, kept muttering, "Oh shit. Oh shit."

Jim finally spoke, well, shouted, "How can this be possible? How can we hire someone who is a self-proclaimed expert in stucco work and have this happen?" He punctuated his question with stabs into the crumbling stucco. "Have this happen?" Stab, scrape, crash. "And this?" Another dust cloud rose around his feet and slabs of stucco fell to the ground.

Frankie didn't answer. He simply shook his head. After a few minutes, he began packing up his gear, and I gave him a tense ride home. As I said goodbye, he said, "Sorry about that," and shut my car door.

I got back home to find Jim beginning the long, sad job of removing the non-sticking stucco from the surface of the house. We worked together, knocking off enormous sheets of the thick, gray rock, watching it crumble on the ground at our feet, and counting the money and time lost as we went. We raked and then bagged it all in construction bags to be hauled off to the dump. Four hours later, we were back where we started, almost. The side of the house was once again it's dull, scraped yellow, but we had learned that the solution needed more bonding agent if it were to adhere properly. Thankfully, we found out before the entire house had been done with the failed stucco solution. Thankfully, we didn't paint it before we found out it would simply fall off if tapped. Thankfully, the mistake was not made in vain.

My second relapse began and ended in the same way as the housework. I thought I was an expert in my addiction, much like Frankie thought he was a stucco expert, even though his only experience was mudding concrete. I believed I could handle it. I knew which boundaries could be pushed, right? Before I knew it, I was relapsing, first in my head, then in my habits, and finally in my eating.

Every Labor Day weekend for years, my husband and I, and later our son, had attended a local festival commemorating the Battle of Fort Henry at the local Revolutionary War-era fort. In addition to the siege, the festival features a period-era settlement, complete with white and Native American actors in full costumes demonstrating activities from daily life in the 1700s, like cooking, spinning wool, blacksmithing, and so on. Of course, period vendors have plenty to sell, including foods. I had eaten before we went, knowing that the chance of finding safe foods at the festival would be incredibly unlikely, but hours later, we were all hungry. As my husband and son quelled their hunger with hot dogs and chips, I wandered into a tent and found roasted corn, which the vendor of the makeshift general store informed me was a staple of the Revolutionary War-era diet, especially among Native Americans.

Since I eat corn regularly, I assumed it would be fine. I took my little bag of kernels back to the table to share with my family. I knew immediately, as I crunched the first kernel, that this snack was dangerous. I should have given them away. Instead, I ate and I ate and I ate. The crunch, the oil, the salt, the sugar starch in the corn. I kept eating and eating, going back twice for more, wiping my slick, salty hands on my pants and ignoring my son's requests for a piggy-back ride, a game of chase, and a walk through of the white muslin tents.

Eventually, the paper bag was empty but for a few specks of salt. I wadded it up and threw it in the trash. Before it even left, the guilt set in, a little admonishment at first, then a wave of crushing self-disappointment.

Why did I take a chance like that?

Why did I think I could handle any food that made my brain flare red hot from the first bite?

I am better than this!

Have I learned nothing in the past year and a half?

In the midst of the self-berating, my son, in a way that only he can, snapped me out of my guilt-laden trance. "Mama, can we take our picture by the big bell?"

I picked him up and hugged him. "Sure, let's do it!"

I look at this photo now, and I see my son and me kneeling by the old camp dinner bell, smiles gleaming, giggling at my husband who was no doubt being goofy behind the camera. It was sunny that day. Hot, like it always is for Fort Henry Days. There is no trace of agony in my face even though I was swimming in the depths of it minutes before.

The roasted corn is only one of the hyper-palatable foods I've tried that have established a hold on me with varying durations. medjool dates, sugar-free hazelnut syrup, and popcorn with olive oil and salt are just some of the foods that made me want to get higher and higher on food.

Like with my lapses and relapses, we made several different attempts at stuccoing our house. Some failed. Some failed miserably. But eventually, my husband found a mixture and application method that worked. It was challenging, physically and mentally, for him as the main laborer and for me as the wife who missed her husband day after day, weekend after weekend as he toiled obsessively with getting it done right.

As he reclaimed the veneer, making it new again with mortar, cementing, bonding, and sand, I once again turned my attention to scraping. This time I was removing decades of thick, cracking paint from the front porch with a heat gun and scraper. My ventilator and glasses protected me from the fumes as the craftsmen red layer bubbled under the 1200 degree heat. I slid my blade beneath the hot goop and slid it off the cornice, revealing, to my surprise, a layer of gun metal grey paint, which I also heated and carefully scraped off. As the gray layer bubbled, I scraped again to discover a startling, grass green layer, which yielded to the heat and pressure to reveal bare wood. It was perfectly preserved oak, hammered in placed almost 80 years ago by workers long since gone, the product of their labor still sound, still solid and still smooth.

My heart leaped a bit when I reached that original layer. I moved my way around our large front porch, knowing that it was possible to strip away years of other peoples' choices, other peoples' ideas. It has been that way for me in recovery as well. Each layer I peel away gets me one step closer to who I am, free of the assumptions of others, free of the toxic haze of being simultaneously overfed and hungry.

Now, every time I see a crack in the paint on a building or along a baseboard in some dark hallway, I long to pick up my scraper and dig away at the looseness, watching with pleasure as chip after chip breaks off and falls away. I no longer see crumbling paint or splintered wood as defects. Like my recovering self, I envision what beauty might lie beneath the flaking façade. I want to peel away the layers to reveal its origins, as rough and hard worn as they may be. I've learned that the true self is desirable, worth uncovering, and I intend to keep scraping.

Epilogue

It came softly. The decades of bitter fighting—me vs. me—were finally over. There was no warning, but no warning was needed. The obsessive thoughts, the compulsive eating, the constant battle to shrink my body and my soul had ceased. Unlike my first day of recovery, I could not mark the moment when it changed. There was no dam break. No sudden bursting of long-standing walls. Instead, it was more like how T. S. Eliot predicts the way the world will end, "Not with a bang but a whimper."

It is difficult to quantify. I don't remember the last time I binged or ate out of boredom or nervousness or dread. I don't remember the last time I thought about one food all day, having memorized its location, flavor, and texture in the way that long-distance lovers might when they feel sudden pangs of lust between visits. I don't remember the last time I craved a food so much that I would drive 25 or more minutes to get it. I don't remember the last time I tore open a container of food in the parking lot of the grocery store to eat, eat, eat it all on the way home.

I am at peace with food. I am at peace with me.

I am not thin. My body is not perfect.

I am at peace with food. I am at peace with me.

I am not recovered. I do not believe in that absolution. All I know is that I have never been here before, and I like it. It is somehow more than serenity, because to me serenity always seemed temporary, like a limbo space we are all dying to get back to or stay in. It is a state of mind, rather than a state of being, because a state of being requires action and is linked to behavior. Instead, I feel that this is my life, my natural state. Three meals a day of whole, nutritious foods. Nothing before. Nothing after. Nothing in between.

This place is far different than I imagined. I do not feel fantastic. I do not feel high or wild with energy. I feel whole. Complete. Essentially sound. Impeccably round. Full. Full of myself. Full of spirit. Full of life being lived now.

I no longer wonder where I will go from here. Will I ever lapse? Will I ever abuse food and myself again? I have no idea. I do not even consider it. If I am lucky, I will have decades of recovery to find out where the road will take me. Until then, I will live each day one day at a time. For the first time, I realize that it can be no other way. Living in the past is a misnomer, an impossibility.

I began recovery optimistic, which was a burden and a blessing, and I have not been disappointed in either case. The manic-depressive days of the first year led to a switch in focus at the beginning of the second, which gradually gave way to my current state: a quiet mind, a full heart, and an open spirit.

My world has changed since the day I stepped off the scale and onto a new path. No day has been the same. No day has been perfect. But every single one has been thoroughly lived. I show up for life, no matter how painful it may be. I show up for life, and the rewards are innumerable.

Other Books
by
Christina Fisanick Greer

Two-Week Wait: Motherhood Lost and Found

The Optimistic Food Addict's Recovery Journal and Activity Book

Select MSI Books

Self-Help Books

57 Steps to Paradise (Lorenz)

A Woman's Guide to Self-Nurturing (Romer)

Creative Aging: A Baby Boomer's Guide to Successful Living (Vassiliadis & Romer)

Divorced! Survival Techniques for Singles over Forty (Romer)

How to Live from Your Heart (Hucknell)

Living Well with Chronic Illness (Charnas)

Publishing for Smarties: Finding a Publisher (Ham)

Survival of the Caregiver (Snyder)

The Rose and the Sword: How to Balance Your Feminine and Masculine Energies (Bach & Hucknall)

The Widower's Guide to a New Life (Romer)

Widow: A Survival Guide for the First Year (Romer)

Inspirational and Religious Books

A Believer-Waiting's First Encounters with God (Mahlou)

A Guide to Bliss: Transforming Your Life through Mind Expansion (Tubali)

El Poder de lo Transpersonal (Ustman)

Everybody's Little Book of Everyday Prayers (MacGregor)

Surviving Cancer, Healing People: One Cat's Story (Sula)

How to Get Happy and Stay That Way: Practical Techniques for Putting Joy into Your Life (Romer)

Joshuanism (Tosto)

Living in Blue Sky Mind (Diedrichs)

Passing On (Romer)

Puertas a la Eternidad (Ustman)

Surviving Cancer, Helping People: One Cat's Story (Sula)

The Gospel of Damascus (O. Imady)

When You're Shoved from the Right, Look to Your Left: Metaphors of Islamic Humanism (O. Imady)

Memoirs

Blest Atheist (Mahlou)

Forget the Goal, the Journey Counts . . . 71 Jobs Later (Stites)

Good Blood, Volume 1 and Volume 2 (Schaffer)

Healing from Incest: Intimate Conversations with My Therapist (Henderson & Emerton)

It Only Hurts When I Can't Run: One Girl's Story (Parker)

Las Historias de Mi Vida (Ustman)

Of God, Rattlesnakes, and Okra (Easterling)

Road to Damascus (E. Imady)

Foreign Culture

Syrian Folktales (M. Imady)

The Rise and Fall of Muslim Civil Society (O. Imady)

The Subversive Utopia: Louis Kahn and the Question of National Jewish Style in Jerusalem (Sakr)

Thoughts without a Title (Henderson)

PSYCHOLOGY & PHILOSOPHY

Anxiety Anonymous: The Big Book on Anxiety Addiction (Ortman)

Depression Anonymous (Ortman)

Road Map to Power (Husain & Husain)

The Marriage Whisperer: How to Improve Your Relationship Overnight (Pickett)

The Seven Wisdoms of Life: A Journey into the Chakras (Tubali)

Understanding the Critic: Socionics in Everyday Life (Quinelle)

Understanding the Entrepreneur: Socionics in Everyday Life (Quinelle)

Understanding the People around You: An Introduction to Socionics (Filatova)

Understanding the Seeker: Socionics in Everyday Life (Quinelle)

HUMOR

How My Cat made Me a Better Man (Feig)

Mommy Poisoned Our House Guest (C. B. Leaver)

The Musings of a Carolina Yankee (Amidon)

PARENTING

365 Teacher Secrets for Parents: Fun Ways to Help Your Child in Elementary School (McKinley & Trombly)

How to Be a Good Mommy When You're Sick (Graves)

Lessons of Labor (Aziz)

CPSIA information can be obtained
at www.ICGtesting.com
Printed in the USA
LVOW01s1451210916
505621LV00016B/595/P

9 781942 891284